THE
POWER
OF
SELF-MANAGEMENT

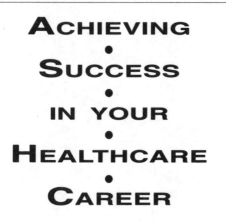

ACHIEVING
•
SUCCESS
•
IN YOUR
•
HEALTHCARE
•
CAREER

by Michael Henry Cohen

 Canoe Press. Oak Park. Illinois

The Power of Self-Management:

Achieving Success in Your Healthcare Career

Word Processing: Diane Dassow
Editing: Nancy Gospo
Book Design: Kate Lanham
Cover Design: Jason Michael Cohen

ISBN 0–9613768–1–3

ABOUT THE AUTHOR

Michael H. Cohen is a nationally recognized workshop leader and consultant, specializing in management development, employee relations, organizational communications, and continuous quality improvement. He has taught Interpersonal Communications, Group Process, and Organizational Behavior at Northwestern University, Roosevelt University and Rosary College and conducts management effectiveness programs for professional associations throughout the United States.

Prior to establishing his consulting practice, Michael served as Director of Employee Relations and Development and Vice President, Human Resources at Weiss Memorial Hospital, Chicago, Illinois for 12 years. He holds a Master of Arts Degree in Communication Studies from Northwestern University and is also the author of the book, *On-The-Job Survival: A Guide for Dealing with Everyday Work Problems.*

Information on Michael H. Cohen's management and employee development workshops can be obtained by writing to:

Michael H. Cohen
Management Consulting Services
333 N. Euclid
Oak Park, IL 60302
(708) 386-1968

ACKNOWLEDGEMENTS

This book is dedicated to the memory of my father, Joseph E. Cohen, who taught me the values of courage, perseverance and fair play; and to the memory of my father-in-law, Chester W. Davey, who taught me the values of service and generosity to family and community.

A Note to the Reader

The "she" pronoun has been used in this book in place of the traditional "he" pronoun when referring to both men and women. This "role-reversal" is more than appropriate given that the majority of healthcare employees are female.

▲

Contents

An institution is the lengthened shadow of one person.

Ralph Waldo Emerson

▲

Chapter 1

INTRODUCTION:

Facing the Human Relations Challenge

The most important individuals working within any healthcare organization are those front-line employees and volunteers who have the most direct and sustained contact with patients, visitors, and physicians. These people are directly responsible for providing a service and maintaining the institution's high-quality reputation.

The vast majority of these employees enjoy the clinical and/or technical aspects of their job, and they are superb in the execution of their duties. What distresses them most, however, is not the *content* of their jobs, but the *context* in which they perform their work. Their underlying job frustrations are caused by a general perception of powerlessness to deal with the human relations challenges and system problems inherent in the working environment. These include:

1. Organizational Politics

Employees comment:

"I'm having trouble making the system work for me. I can't get the support from 'higher-ups' or secure the resources I need to get my job done."

"Why can't the people at the top understand what's going on at *our* level? Why doesn't anyone check with us first before making a decision? Why doesn't anyone utilize our expertise? We're on the front lines, making things happen. We're handling the complaints and answering the challenging questions; we know what will work and what won't work. I try telling them, but they won't listen."

2. The Verbally Abusive Physician

Employees comment:

"I shouldn't have to put up with a doctor who constantly insults and humiliates me, who talks down to me in a condescending manner as if I'm a child in need of a lecture, in full public view of patients, visitors and co-workers. I have the right to defend myself against this tyrannical behavior. However, if I am assertive, will I get support from hospital administration?"

3. A Lazy or Incompetent Co-Worker

Employees comment:

"I have to work side by side with a prima donna. She is overbearing and intimidating. She may be technically competent and clinically sound, but her style of addressing problems is creating defensiveness and hostility on the unit. She's raising havoc on group morale and productivity. I'm trying to resist getting sucked into the conflict, but I don't know what to do."

"We have this nasty conflict between the day and evening shift. A huge breakdown in communication and cooperation has developed. Patient care is falling through the cracks. The staff is polarized and we can't seem to iron out the differences."

4. Managerial Malpractice

Employees comment:

"My boss is unpredictable. She's subject to extreme mood swings. I never know how she's going to react from one minute to the next. So I have to be cautious in my communications with her."

"My boss is quick to criticize me when I make a mistake, but rarely, if ever, do I hear a compliment for the good work I do (which is most of the time). Because the only feedback I seem to get is negative, I simply try to avoid her as much as possible."

"Why doesn't my manager do something about this lazy, incompetent co-worker of ours? By doing nothing, she's sending out a signal to the rest of us that her behavior is acceptable. In the meantime, we all are working harder to compensate for her deficiency, and we resent it bitterly."

5. Inability to Personally Cope

Employees comment:

"I'm having a real difficult time dealing with all the changes going on around here. Every time I turn around someone is being laid off, a program is being dropped, or a new service is being added. We're constantly putting out fires. The pressures are intense, and the stress never seems to let up. While we're short-staffed, management is asking us to work harder and faster. We're beginning to compromise on professional standards to meet the impossible demands. And to add insult to injury, we're being told to smile all the time!"

6. Dramatic Shift in Organizational Culture

Employees comment:

"I used to feel as if we were one large family. Everybody looked out for and supported one another. I don't see that any more. We're always being told that the hospital is a 'business.' Each department is seen as a 'cost center.' We either produce revenue or represent overhead. It seems the only thing administration is interested in is the bottom line. We're not even supposed to call patients 'patients' anymore. They're now 'customers' or 'guests.' But this is not a *hotel*, it's a hospital. We have a special kind of relationship with our patients, and I resent the comparison with other industries. If this is the wave of the future, I'm not sure I want to be a part of it."

Added to these problems is the inherent stress of the healthcare environment. Patient care is an emotionally intensive and physically exhausting activity. Healthcare employees face stress and conflict when dealing with the upset or demanding patient or visitor, when negotiating with difficult co-workers and bosses, and when trying to access resources from other shifts and departments.

Achieving satisfaction and success is possible under all of the above scenarios, but it requires fairly sophisticated, yet common sense skills in communication, problem solving and conflict management. These skills when used consistently, add up to *self-management*: the ability to manage one's own feelings and act constructively within a stressful, fast-paced and highly competitive work environment. Utilizing self-management skills and possessing the ability to adapt to conditions beyond one's control are critical to career success.

Management's Role

At present, most schools and healthcare institutions do not adequately prepare employees for the realities of the work place. As a result, far too many employees are leaving the profession because of their inability to handle the human relations challenges inherent in their jobs. If hospitals and other healthcare institutions are to succeed in retaining these highly qualified and well-motivated employees, they must empower employees with the ability and the authority to independently solve problems and manage interpersonal conflicts. They must also provide employees with the necessary freedom, autonomy and control over their own working environment so that employees feel vested in their work.

Booker T. Washington said, "Few things help individuals more than to place responsibility upon them, and let them know that you trust them." Abraham Lincoln said, "You cannot help people permanently by doing for them what they could and should do for themselves." Most employees want the opportunity to independently carry out their work responsibilities without their manager hovering over them. They would also prefer to resolve everyday problems without deferring to management all of the time. They sincerely want what is best for the hospital and its patients, and they are willing to do what is necessary to achieve desired outcomes. In short, the vast majority of employees *want* to be self-managed. They do, however, expect their manager to give direction, provide resources that set them up for success, act as an organizational ally, and remove the systems barriers that impede the accomplishment of their goals. Assuming the manager meets these expectations, most employees recognize that they are responsible and accountable for the results of their efforts.

In addition, management needs to take an active role in providing employees with effective stress management and conflict management skills. These skills will enable employees to solve everyday work problems at the earliest (and lowest) levels so they don't have to defer to management at each instance for resolution of difficulties. If all employees understood how to effectively negotiate interpersonal conflicts, it would improve the quality of organizational decisions, the speed with which problems are resolved, and the level of cooperation between various sectors within the hospital.

Preparing employees for self-management, then, will facilitate success in handling the difficult human relations challenges inherent within the healthcare organization. It will also improve the overall quality of service because employees will feel more responsible for identifying and constructively addressing technical and customer relations issues.

A self-managed employee is an employee who is committed to the success of the organization and who has mastered those technical and interpersonal skills necessary to achieve positive results. This book has been written, therefore, to help employees understand this powerful concept of self-management and practice it in their everyday work lives.

Notes:

Every man's work
is a portrait of himself.

Anonymous

---▲---

Chapter 2

WHY SELF-MANAGEMENT?

This book focuses on self-management as a strategy for successfully dealing with on-the-job stress, change, and interpersonal conflict. It is designed to empower you with effective communication and conflict-management skills that will make your job easier, more satisfying and effective. Self-management calls for you to tolerate the common frustrations that are a natural part of your job. When you practice self-management, you accept the limitations of your boss and fellow employees, and you learn how to get understanding and cooperation from them so that your work is more effective as well as pleasant.

When you practice self-management you demonstrate:

1. Flexibility and Adaptability

You are not paralyzed by change. You are able to adjust to an increasingly fast-paced, highly-competitive and constantly changing work environment.

2. Versatility

You make yourself more valuable when you are willing to learn new skills and apply them to organizational needs. You demonstrate versatility when you accept criticism non-defensively and experiment with new behaviors that lead to personal growth.

3. High Tolerance for Ambiguity

In the midst of change and uncertainty, you don't wait for your marching orders. You take the initiative and act affirmatively. You focus on those things that are within your control and do the very best you can, thereby creating your own structure and positive spheres of influence.

4. Respect for Differences of Opinion

You effectively manage conflicts, always maintaining integrity and respect for yourself and others. You do this by addressing issues in a collaborative and constructive manner rather than personally attacking a co-worker with whom you are in disagreement.

5. Excitement About New Possibilities

You view change as a challenge and a new opportunity for growth and contribution to the organization. You don't look back to the "good old days" because things will never be the same. As Tom Wolfe said, "You can never go home again."

6. Responsibility

You understand that you are ultimately responsible for your own success and happiness on the job, and that attaining the good life on the job is not an inalienable right. There are no guarantees for job security or entitlements for job fulfillment. To succeed, therefore, you must take personal responsibility and hold yourself accountable for effective work performance.

7. Pursuit of Excellence

You acknowledge that your number one objective on the job is to be successful, not happy. Happiness on the job is usually a by-product of success. Happiness comes from taking pride in your work. It comes from being a part of a successful team effort. Happiness comes from observing the positive results of your effort. Regardless of work constraints and limitations, your primary focus is always on the contribution that you are making on behalf of the patient.

8. Realistic Expectations

You understand that there exists no perfect working environment, free of frustrations or irritations. Therefore, you take full advantage of the positive aspects of the job, try to improve those things that are within your control to change, and adjust to those things you can't change. You remain flexible in your dealings with patients, managers and co-workers.

9. Effective Boss Relationships

You accept the fact that you don't have to like your boss on a personal level in order to have an effective working relationship. Of course, it's nicer and easier to work with a boss you like, but it's not a pre-condition for a successful working relationship. The best boss in the world cannot make you successful, and the worst boss cannot make you fail. You always have choices to make regarding where and for whom you are going to work. But if you choose to stay, your number one priority is to secure a harmonious working relationship with the boss. Successful employees, in fact, "manage the boss" as effectively as the boss manages them. And if you want to be managed less by your boss, you have to manage yourself more.

10. Self-Motivation

You realize that even the most talented boss cannot motivate you to do an outstanding job. She can, on occasion, de-motivate you through a litany of management sins. But she cannot motivate you. Motivation has to come from within and is the product of your own work ethic. As a self-managed employee, you approach the job with a strong sense of commitment that demonstrates:

- "I'm able to work as the schedule requires on a consistent basis. You can count on me to be here. I am reliable."

- "I'm willing to put in a hard day's work for an honest day's pay. I will take the initiative and follow through on tasks to successful completion. I am independent and self-directed."

- "I feel good when I do something nice for someone. I enjoy serving others, and I will go the extra mile to ensure that I fully meet (or exceed) their expectations."

This work ethic is based upon your personal values established long before you ever entered the work world. It was developed during your formative years when you were learning the values of responsibility, team work, completing what you started, and honoring your commitments. This work ethic is intrinsic; if you don't possess it, even the best manager will find it difficult to motivate you.

Your manager's job is to effectively select personnel who possess these work values from the start, lead by example, provide recognition and reward for achievement, and create a positive work environment that *facilitates* your success. If you possess the technical skills, creativity and desire to succeed, your manager can channel this energy toward constructive ends consistent with a common vision. But she cannot *make* you successful. That's your responsibility. No matter how inspiring or charismatic your manager may be, she cannot light a fire beneath you unless you provide the initial spark or will to achieve. Self-managed employees are, in effect, self-motivated employees.

If you make yourself dependent upon someone else for your own motivation and professional success, you place your job effectiveness and satisfaction in a vulnerable position, dependent upon external forces outside your control. Others have to like you or approve of your work in order for you to feel secure. You must get the attention or credit you deserve, otherwise you will feel cheated. Your boss must be all knowing, nurturing, attentive, consistent, and appreciative (be everything you ever wanted in a parent), or else you feel cheated. But your boss can never be everything that you want her to be. More important, your boss cannot give you your freedom, your self-esteem, or sense of security. That's *your* life's task.

If your desire is to work in an organization that makes you feel safe and protected, the price you pay for it is dependency. You will be dependent on your boss or the "system" to take care of you. But in the real world, there are no guarantees of job security and there are no entitlements for job fulfillment. Likewise, if you truly want freedom in your job, the price you pay is accountability, knowing that only *you* are responsible for your own job happiness and success, that you always have choices available in response to work conflicts and that you are always accountable for the results of your decisions.

There is no safety in self-management and autonomy, but self-management is what's required to be successful and satisfied on the job. Of course, independence and autonomy are not to be pursued for their own sake. Autonomy without a higher purpose is self-serving and only leads to anarchy. As a self-managed employee, you claim your autonomy in service to a vision and set of values. You decide, "I'm here to serve, to contribute, to do something that has meaning." Good bosses and co-workers can help you in this endeavor, but they are not the answer to your search for meaning, value and integrity at work.

▲

Self-Management is Motivated Primarily by Intrinsic Rewards

Intrinsic motivation encourages the employee to enjoy work because the activity is enjoyable and meaningful as well as a source of income. When the motivation is essentially extrinsic, the terms of achievement are imposed from outside oneself and are, therefore, outer-directed.[1]

When Motivation is Extrinsic or Outer-Directed	*When Motivation is Intrinsic or Self-Directed*
The employee's desire is fueled by the pursuit of material rewards, praise, or recognition.	The employee's desire is fueled by passion, pride, and a responsible work ethic.
The employee is preoccupied with the performance of boss, co-workers and organizational politics.	The employee's primary concern is being the best she can be and making a significant contribution regardless how others act.
Hard work or challenging situations are resented by the employee for the amount of extra energy and time required to complete the task.	Hard work or challenging situations are not regarded as a personal sacrifice, because the employee "owns her job" and wants to follow through to achieve positive results.

When Motivation is Extrinsic or Outer-Directed	When Motivation is Intrinsic or Self-Directed
The employee's focus is on competition, getting credit, and on "looking good" in comparison with others.	The employee's focus is on personal and professional fulfillment. The job itself is highly valued and has meaning in the employee's life.
External success (raises, promotions, job security, prestige, adulation) is largely determined or provided by others.	Intrinsic success (signaled by high self-esteem, pride, and enthusiasm) is largely determined by the employee.
The pursuit of external success can easily lead to workaholism and burnout at the expense of personal fulfillment. Work can become all consuming and exhausting.	The pursuit of intrinsic success usually leads to a healthy balance between personal and work life because the employee is in touch with her own feelings and values.

Self-Management Requires
High Self-Esteem

Characteristics of employees with high self-esteem are:

- People who pronounce a self-verdict or self-judgement that indicates, "I have personal power and competence. I intend to work in a fulfilling and personally meaningful way."

- People who are "psychologically" successful within themselves and possess *inner affluence.* Regardless of their level or role within the organization, their underlying belief is that they are living out life's purpose through their own effort and creative will. This inner vision and sense of mission is the primary source of overcoming any obstacle (internal or external). They are able to find something in any assignment that brings them a sense of satisfaction and accomplishment.

- People who possess a moral code of conduct, values, ethics, and personal laws to live by. They are not motivated by external injunctions so much as a belief in themselves and what they stand for.

- People who believe that they are not put on earth to struggle through life. They don't weigh themselves down with the heavy baggage of fear, guilt or other self-defeating thought patterns. They also don't blame others when faced with everyday work frustrations that inhibit their job success or happiness.

- People who are self-disciplined and are willing to take the time and effort to get what they want. They solve problems creatively and assertively and act from a base of self-trust. Their self-statements tell them that they have what it takes to figure out what to do when faced with any adversity.

- People who don't hope for someone else to do difficult chores for them or rescue them from the tedious, demanding tasks at hand. They take responsibility to do what needs to be done to accomplish a goal or satisfy a need. They place a great reliance upon themselves, therefore, in determining the course of their work lives.

- People who follow the often slow and difficult path of self-discipline, perseverance and integrity. Regardless of job constraints and limitations, they remain generally enthusiastic, focused and purposeful.

continued...

Self-Management Requires High Self-Esteem

Characteristics of employees with high self-esteem are:

- People who are able to tell others what they need, feel, or want in a plain-spoken, forthright, and respectful way. They have successfully faced the challenge of learning how to be treated well.

- People who are able and willing to take risks and move into the unknown. These risks, however, are not taken blindly. They are well planned and typically produce beneficial outcomes. They mentally rehearse and visualize what might happen. They identify their options and then put one hundred percent energy into making the decision or action successful.

- People who allow their weaknesses to be worked on, while their strengths and talents grow into full use. They are in continuous pursuit of self-improvement yet are able to acknowledge and take pride in who they are and what they have already accomplished.

- People who consciously *choose* to do their work and accept the rewards and consequences for this choice. They cultivate self-respect and inner security by ultimately holding themselves responsible for their own job success and happiness.

Notes:

One thing I know; the only ones among you who will be really happy are those who will have sought and found how to serve.

Albert Schweitzer

▲

Chapter 3

THE IMPORTANCE OF PEOPLE SKILLS

Healthcare is a service industry, and as an employee, the care or service you render to patients and visitors is your particular product. Service as a product, however, is vastly different from the manufacturing of "tangible" products such as automobiles. Cars are manufactured and checked for quality inside and out before placed on the showroom floor. There are various checkpoints in the manufacturing process to minimize mistakes. Service as a product, however, is manufactured at the instant of delivery. It has to be right the first time. There is no second chance to create a positive first impression.

Every time a patient or visitor comes in contact with you, there is a "moment of truth" in the delivery of your service. With every encounter, you are transacting business and projecting a corporate image. And the sum of every encounter a person has with you adds up to her overall evaluation of your quality of service. For each patient or visitor, there must be many such "moments of truth" during the day, and each time, you are being tested for your genuine level of interest.

It is also important to remember that the patient or visitor is motivated by her own particular needs and expectations. She is not necessarily loyal to your hospital. Therefore, if you want to gain the patient's voluntary compliance, you must first view her as a consumer who has a choice to willingly accept or reject the services you offer. This requires building a relationship of trust and open communications, of establishing your personal and professional credibility.

Service is inherently a perception issue. That is, if the customer (a patient, visitor, or employee requiring your service) does not *perceive* she has been served well, then by definition, she has *not* been served well. Quality is whatever the customer says it is. You don't define it, the customer does, based upon her own subjective criteria.

The customer's perceptions, right or wrong, are always *real*, and you have to deal with those perceptions as reality. If, for example, a patient's expectations of you are unrealistic, you still have to legitimize these expectations, then educate and/or negotiate with the patient to get her perceptions in line with "reality." This requires sophisticated communication skills and a non-judgmental approach to difficult patients. After all, your job is not to *judge* the patient. Your job is to *serve* her. And you can't do both very well at the same time.

For a service-oriented employee, there is no such thing as a "good customer" or a "bad customer." Some people may be more challenging than others, but as soon as you label the customer, you lose the objective psychological distance needed to effectively serve the individual. Service calls for your *unconditional* acceptance of a customer's perceptions or expectations and your willingness to deal with the person as she naturally presents herself to you. It is counterproductive to respond judgmentally based on some pre-conditioned notion of how the customer *should* be behaving.

As a healthcare employee, you are not going to be judged by your *intent* to do well or by how hard you try. You're going to be evaluated by *results*, by the impact you have on others, and by the impressions you make as a representative of your organization. You can't measure "intent." You can, however, measure results or verify the impact that one person has on another. And in healthcare, your human relations skills often have a greater impact on the customer's perception of quality than your technical or clinical skills.

Most patients or visitors are not experts on the technical or clinical aspects of your job. They *assume* that you are technically competent or else you wouldn't be employed within the healthcare institution. Your clinical expertise is a *given* for them. Furthermore, most patients and visitors are not able to distinguish one employee from another based upon levels of competence. Their evaluation of employees is made based upon employees' communications and human relations skills, not clinical skills. In fact, you can make a technical mistake, and if you catch it in time, the average patient will never know the difference. But all patients and visitors are experts on whether they are being treated with empathy, courtesy and respect, regardless of their sophistication or technical knowledge.

Patient opinion surveys consistently report the same findings: When a discharged patient feels that employees were unpleasant, she gives the hospital very low marks on the perceived quality of care. She says negative things about the hospital even though she improved physically. On the other hand, when a patient feels that employees were kind and compassionate, she gives the hospital very high marks on the perceived quality of care. She says good things about the hospital even if she did *not* improve physically. These findings confirm that an employee's human relations skills, and an ability to communicate through words and gestures that, "I really care for you," are as important as clinical skills.

Comparisons with other industries are always dangerous because the healthcare industry is unique, but my experience with airlines may be illustrative here. Frankly, I would not choose to get on an airplane unless I made two sets of assumptions. The first assumption regards the pilot. I have to believe that he is technically competent. He is not a substance abuser. He does not suffer from an acute state of depression or harbor a secret death wish. He has had a good night's sleep. In short, he is fully capable of navigating the plane.

The second assumption that I make before getting on the airplane, is that the ground crew has made the craft airworthy. No defective bolts have been used. All parts have been securely fastened. The engines have been thoroughly checked and are operating properly. I simply want to feel confident that the airplane is completely safe for successful take-off and landing. I wouldn't endanger my life unless I believed in the technical skills of the airline employees and the safety of the aircraft.

As a consumer, I am not in a position to differentiate one airline carrier from another based upon technical criteria. The airline companies know this. When they run a television commercial, the message to the public is *not*, "Fly United Airlines... we have a better *crash record* than American!" Of course not. Instead, United Airlines asks potential customers to, "Fly the Friendly Skies," attempting to convey a warm and compassionate image. Delta Airlines counters with, "We Love to Fly and It Shows," implying that their employees enjoy their jobs and are eager to please the customers.

Today, hospitals are equally engaged in high-stakes competition, and are attempting to project in the public eye the same friendly image. When a hospital runs a full-page advertisement in the local newspaper, it doesn't say, "Come to Community Hospital... We Have a Lower *Death Rate* than Memorial Hospital!" Of course not. It's more likely to say, "Come to Memorial Hospital: We Care For You." Hospitals, like airlines, understand that purchases of service are made based upon perceptions of friendliness and convenience, not technical skills.

It wasn't always this way in the healthcare industry. Not too many years ago, the only competition hospitals experienced consisted of physicians vying with one another to get their patients admitted into the hospital. Census levels were relatively high, the average length of stay was up, and patient acuity levels were reasonable. Most hospitals were virtual gold mines. Money was being made hand over fist. It really didn't matter from a financial perspective whether a patient felt good about the quality of his stay at the hospital. After all, there were more than enough patients to occupy the beds.

During the 1980's, however, census levels began to drop. With the advent of D.R.G.'s, patient acuity levels got higher and length of stays got shorter. Today, hospitals can't *afford* to have patients leaving the hospital feeling that they were "treated badly" by employees. This negative perception is a real threat to the hospital's economic well-being. In fact, a patient who has a negative experience in the hospital will tell *seven times as many people* than a patient who has a favorable stay. This kind of negative publicity can literally destroy the reputation of a healthcare institution.

In response to the challenge, hospitals across the country have instituted "guest relations" and continuous quality improvement programs for the purpose of making employees more sensitive to the service aspects of their jobs. In many hospitals, improved monitoring and evaluation systems have been established to analyze patient perceptions. New recognition strategies have been developed to reward service-oriented employees. Policies and procedures have been audited to determine if they are "user-friendly," and programs have been initiated to facilitate improved communication and coordination between departments.

Practicing outstanding patient and visitor relations is no longer an employee *choice*. It is a condition of employment. There is a bottom-line expectation within hospitals that effective communications are to be exhibited even under the most stressful situations. This service-management concept is being operationalized through performance appraisals and disciplinary actions. Merit increases and continued employment status hinge on the demonstration of employees' human relations and service management skills. Customer-focused standards are being built into the evaluation process with the expectation that:

1. The employee is able to identify more than one solution or alternative for dealing with resistant patients or visitors.

2. The employee will invest considerable time developing trust, establishing personal credibility and determining the unique needs of the patient.

3. The employee will demonstrate an understanding that the personal relationship she develops with the patient greatly influences her ability to render quality care. Therefore, she must be attentive to the various little things that can be done to convey interest and care.

4. The employee will "hustle" for the patient. Hustle is demonstrated by more than a quick pace. It is evident in follow-through, enthusiasm, and a delivery of service that exceeds (not just meets) patient expectations. Hustle is any action that communicates, "I'm working on your behalf. I will jockey the system, if necessary, to make it work for you. I have your best interests in mind."

5. The employee truly gets a kick out of doing something nice for patients and visitors, and it shows through both verbal and non-verbal behavior.

The Importance of Effective Employee Relations

The need for displaying outstanding human relations is not limited to patient and visitor relationships. Managing various conflicts with co-workers, within and between departments, shifts, job classifications and, of course, with your boss is also an art form requiring sensitive and sophisticated communication skills.

You can't possibly *like* everyone with whom you work on an equal basis. But whether you are personal friends with a co-worker or not, maintaining an effective working relationship with her will make your job easier, more satisfying and effective. If a colleague does something that frustrates you or impedes your ability to get your job done, you must talk to her about it directly, honestly and respectfully. Instead of raising the person's defensiveness, you must address the issue in a collaborative manner, behind closed doors, within the spirit of confidentiality and non-competitiveness. During the confrontation, you must level *with* the person, not *level* the person.

As a self-managed employee, you don't use personal dislikes as an excuse for maintaining counter-productive working relationships. Regardless of the nature or scope of the conflict, you realize that the hospital's mission of achieving high quality patient care transcends your turf battles. Regardless of personal feelings toward one another, your work roles are interdependent: your job begins, ends, and overlaps with hers in some fashion. Therefore, it is critical that you cooperate and help each other look good in the eyes of the patient. You may never be the best of pals with this co-worker, and some of your conflicts may never be resolved. But if the conflict can't be resolved, it certainly must be effectively *managed* or patient care will suffer.

Maintaining positive working relationships with co-workers you don't personally like is not a compromise on your integrity, nor does it mean you're being a phony. What it suggests is that you pick your fights with discretion and maintain a functional coexistence with the person. You don't allow a breakdown in the relationship. You play the role of a good "organizational citizen," cooperating with each other as the job dictates.

In the last analysis, working in a hospital is a *performing art.* You are always on stage. You can never let your guard down or break character. This is not easy. There are days when you don't feel like "going on." You have a headache or a personal problem. You are upset about a management decision, or your anger is directed toward another department that is not producing in a timely manner. You're tired from lack of sleep or an exhausting schedule. How do you consistently maintain a professional image, respond positively to these challenges, and remain self-managed? The answer to this question is found in your ability to handle the human relations challenges of the job, recognizing that you can never be successful and satisfied at work until you learn how to:

1.   Adjust to the imperfections in others and adapt to problems that can't be changed.

2.   Negotiate in good faith with patients, visitors, and co-workers to secure win-win outcomes.

3.   Establish a sound and secure working relationship with your boss.

4.   Receive and accept criticism in a non-defensive manner.

5.   Learn to package your ideas to win support of influential people within your organization.

6.   Establish personal and professional credibility, acquire the image of a person who possesses practical knowledge, reflects high character and demonstrates good will toward others.

Each of these skills focuses upon the importance of effective human relations as a pre-condition to your job success and satisfaction.

▲

Notes:

He who has never learned to
follow can never lead.
He who has never learned to
obey can never command.

Aristotle

▲

Chapter 4

COLLABORATING WITH YOUR BOSS

If you are self-managed, you will take complete responsibility for your own job success and satisfaction. This includes taking responsibility for choosing a reasonable, competent boss with whom you can establish an effective working relationship. Can you adapt to your boss' style? Is your immediate working environment conducive to job satisfaction? Is the job itself still challenging or interesting enough for you to stay?

You should periodically conduct a personal and professional audit to assess your job satisfaction and commitment to the organization that employs you. Here are the critical issues to address as you audit your work:

1. Pay and Benefits

Do you consider the compensation and benefit package fair, given the amount of effort required to do the job? How does the package compare with that of your peers employed within the organization when you consider the amount of work they have or how well they perform? How does the package compare with employees in *other* healthcare organizations or industries engaged in jobs requiring comparable education and experience?

2. Work Environment

Do you work with people you like and respect? Do you share a common vision and values? Are your recognition needs (praise, status, respect) being met? Do you enjoy opportunities for professional growth? Are you achieving results that are fulfilling? Do you experience the appropriate amount of autonomy (freedom, independence and control) over your immediate working environment? Is your boss responsive to your needs?

3. Job Content

Do you enjoy the actual tasks in which you are engaged? How much effort is required to be successful? What are the psychological or physical costs involved? Is the effort worth it in relation to the rewards? Can you achieve the results that are expected? Are these expectations too easily attained, thereby not challenging or stimulating? Are the expectations too challenging or almost impossible to meet?

4. Consequences

Are you presently on a collision-course with your boss? Do you agree with the majority of her decisions? Can you live with her management style? Do you enjoy following her lead? How important are the negative consequences if you don't do what's expected? Will you receive a marginal performance appraisal? Disciplinary action? Discharge? How badly do you want or need this job? What are your alternatives? What are the risks if you try something else? What are the risks if you *don't* try something else?

Remember, you are not captive or victim to your work situation unless you choose to be. Powerlessness is a self-imposed condition. If you are miserable in your job or indignant about your manager's style, understand that no one has you locked and chained to your present job. As a self-managed employee, it is your responsibility to make career decisions that are self-promoting and conducive to job fulfillment.

One of the most critical determinants of your job success and satisfaction is the working relationship that you establish with your manager. As a self-managed employee, it is as much *your* responsibility as it is your supervisor's to create and maintain a harmonious and productive working relationship. If you are experiencing difficulty with your boss, it is best to examine what *you* can do, not what you can get your boss to do. And, a large part of successfully "managing your boss" is understanding that she can do only so much to provide for your job satisfaction. She has her own job to do in addition to her employee relations responsibilities. Therefore, you need to maintain realistic expectations regarding her ability to satisfy your needs. You also must legitimize her responsibility to make difficult and, when necessary, unpopular decisions.

Profile of the Effective Manager

The best managers are almost always demanding managers, provided they recognize and reward achievement and act as effective role models for the behavior they expect in employees. They lead by example. They work hard and accomplish their own tasks in a timely and effective manner. They practice effective human relations particularly under stressful situations.

But while the outstanding manager embraces these high standards for herself, she also holds all employees accountable for outstanding results consistent with her vision and set of work values. She wants her department to "stand for" something, and she identifies a few critical objectives that she is willing to go to any length to accomplish. These objectives become the central focus of her attention. She spends a considerable amount of time discussing and planning around them, constantly reminding employees that outstanding results are important.

The effective manager also establishes high standards and evaluates employee performance against these standards. She demonstrates a willingness to stretch employees to greater levels of productivity and interpersonal sensitivity. Her expectations are high, and the burden is always placed on the employee to meet each of these expectations providing:

1. The expectation is *job-related* based upon business necessity. It falls within the letter or spirit of your job description and is consistent with your department's overall objectives.

2. The expectation is *achievable*: Other employees facing similar constraints and limitations have been able to perform as expected. Therefore, it is reasonable to assume you can also achieve the desired result.

3. The expectation has been *communicated to you in advance.* You are not being held accountable for something you didn't know about. You have been made aware of this specific responsibility as well as the rewards and consequences for achieving (or not achieving) it.

4. The expectation *is not a threat to your personal safety,* nor does it require actions on your part that are unethical or compromising.

5. The expectation is *consistently and fairly enforced* without regard to your race, national origin, religion, sex, age or disability.

If your manager's expectations meet the above criteria, it becomes your responsibility to perform the task. You have to decide if you will meet your manager's expectations or, when possible, negotiate an acceptable alternative. Knowing the rewards or consequences that await you, the final choice is always yours.

The Nature of Commitments

Every time you agree to do something, you are, in effect, saying to your manager, "Regardless of external forces (foreseen and unforeseen), I will make good on this commitment. You can depend on me." You are reflecting a clear and strong intent that you will do whatever it takes to produce the desired result.

When you make this agreement, the implication is that you have already assessed the potential road blocks and limited resources, but you will not be governed by them. You have looked at the external facts and conditions that exist or that may occur in the future and you have determined that you can deal with whatever comes up. In short, you are creating an island of certainty in an uncertain and unpredictable world.

Once you commit to something, as a self-managed employee, you do what you said you were going to do within the agreed-upon time frame. You simply don't agree to do something unless you believe the circumstances will allow you to honor the commitment and that you truly intend to follow through to successful completion. If you are unsure about your ability to succeed, you negotiate *up front*, rather than renege on the agreement later.

If you ever agree to something and later discover that unforeseen conditions prevent you from accomplishing the objective, it is then incumbent upon you to immediately re-negotiate the agreement. But this re-negotiation cannot be unilateral. The extenuating circumstances should be discussed as soon as they surface, with you and your manager agreeing to a new set of arrangements. If you don't keep her informed of the obstacles which prevent you from honoring the original agreement, and you make excuses after the fact, trust in the relationship breaks down. Your credibility diminishes.

It is your professional responsibility within this working relationship to make informed decisions that are self-promoting and that lead to positive results. It is also your responsibility to recognize all of the constructive choices available to you in response to disagreements with your manager. The choices you make during these occasions will largely determine your job success and satisfaction. The following chapters will discuss in more depth the power of choice in your work life and will describe four specific options available to you when faced with on-the-job frustrations.

▲

Managing Your Boss

You should consider it a number one priority to secure a harmonious working relationship with your boss. Successful employees "manage their boss" as effectively as the boss manages them. How well do you manage your boss? Use the checklist below to find out.

Do you keep your cool when your boss criticizes your work?

YES ___ **No** ___

Comment:
Nobody's perfect. You need feedback to let you know how you're coming across to others and to identify areas for development. Even if you believe your boss is wrong, her perceptions are real, and the burden is on you to change those perceptions.

Do you hope and expect your boss will mess up and secretly delight when she does?

YES ___ **No** ___

Comment:
Part of your job is to help make your boss look good and to set her up for success. By doing so, your boss will be more willing to facilitate your success and satisfaction on the job or be more forgiving when you make a mistake.

Do you play public win-lose games with your boss?

YES ___ No ___

Comment:

When you openly go toe-to-toe with the boss, the smart money bets with the boss almost every time. Besides, all disagreements should be aired behind closed doors in the spirit of confidentiality and non-competitiveness.

Do you bad-mouth your boss behind her back?

YES ___ No ___

Comment:

This practice almost always comes back to haunt you. Remember the time-proven principle, "If you don't have something good to say about someone, it's better not to say anything at all."

Do you expect perfection from your boss?

YES ___ No ___

Comment:

If you do, you will be disappointed. Your manager is a human being subject to flaws like everyone else. Maximize her strengths and minimize her weaknesses.

continued...

Managing Your Boss

...continued

Do you keep your manager informed when something goes wrong?

Yes ___ **N**o ___

Comment:

Managers hate to trip over problems or find out about them from someone outside the department when you had ample opportunity to inform her about the fact. Cover-ups are often worse than the error itself. Likewise, you can't expect the boss to understand your job constraints and limitations unless you keep open the lines of communication.

Do you sanction and legitimize your boss' right to coach and counsel, make out schedules and assignments, and take corrective actions as necessary?

Yes ___ **N**o ___

Comment:

It's the law of organizational life that everyone is accountable to someone. When you accepted the job, you signed your name to an unwritten psychological contract that you will accept and respect your manager's position and cooperate with her, regardless of your personal feelings.

**Do you empathize with your boss'
pressures, job frustrations,
insecurities, etc.?**

YES ___ NO ___

Comment:
If you are sensitive to your boss' needs and expectations, she will probably be more understanding of yours.

**Do you volunteer to do work that
goes beyond your job description?**

YES ___ NO ___

Comment:
Displaying initiative and going the extra mile shows that you have the best interests of the organization in mind, which casts a positive reflection on you.

**Do you insist on having it "your
way or no way?"**

YES ___ NO ___

Comment:
One of the principles of job survival is knowing when to "go to the mat" on disagreements and knowing when to "go with the flow." When you constantly demand changes from your boss, you invite defensiveness and resistance. Pick your fights with discretion.

continued...

Managing Your Boss

...continued

Do you give positive feedback to your boss when deserved?

YES ___ No ___

Comment:

Whenever your boss does something that you really appreciate, by all means acknowledge it. The positive feedback must be sincere and appropriate or it will be viewed as a cheap gimmick.

Do you utilize your boss as a valued resource to facilitate your success?

YES ___ No ___

Comment:

Request your manager's assistance and involvement in areas of her particular interest or expertise. Likewise, demonstrate independence and self-initiative in areas of work in which your manager is *not* strong.

Do you truly demonstrate self-management?

YES ___ No ___

Comment:

The old-fashioned American Work Ethic of putting in a hard day's work for an honest day's pay still makes sense. When you work hard, the day goes by faster and there is a real sense of pride from doing the best job you can.

Are you using your boss as an excuse for being ineffective or unhappy?

Yes ___ No ___

Comment:

It is each employee's responsibility to find success and satisfaction on the job. The best boss can't make you successful, and the worst boss can't make you fail. When faced with a serious problem, remember your options. Becoming a gripe and dumper almost always guarantees frustration and failure.

Do you really understand why you're on the payroll and appreciate the importance of doing a good job?

Yes ___ No ___

Comment:

Your job, regardless of title or status, is critical to the success of the organization, otherwise the position wouldn't exist. In the last analysis, what you *do* for a living is not as important as *how* you do it. Professional success or happiness does not spring from your placement on the organizational chart. It generates from enjoying your work and taking pride in your accomplishments.

Notes:

He who does not make a choice
makes a choice.

Anonymous

▲

Chapter 5

THE POWER OF CHOICE

You're never captive or powerless on the job unless you *choose* to be. The perception of captivity and powerlessness is self-imposed and is always disabling. Eleanor Roosevelt once observed, "No one can hurt you without your consent." Mahatma Gandhi said, "No one can take away your self-respect if you do not give it to them." It's your willing permission or consent that helps or hurts you far more than external forces over which you have no control.

Viktor Frankl, a Jewish psychiatrist who was imprisoned in a Nazi concentration camp, illustrates the powerful dimension of choice even under the worst of human circumstances.[2] Frankl's entire family, with the exception of his sister, perished in the camps. He lost every material possession, suffered from hunger, cold and brutality. Stripped to his naked existence, he faced potential hourly extermination.

In the concentration camp, every circumstance conspired to make him lose hold of his basic human values. All of the familiar goals in his life were snatched away. But what remained for Frankl was the "last of human freedoms," the ability to "choose one's attitude in a given set of circumstances." Throughout this horrific experience, Frankl chose to maintain a sense of meaning and responsibility in his existence.

Without question, the camps facilitated a strong feeling among the prisoners that fate was their only master and that one must not try to influence it in any way. The temptation was overwhelming to allow the environment to completely dictate one's attitudes and behavior. But within this context, Frankl dared to ask:

> "But what about human liberty? Is there no spiritual freedom in regard to behavior and reaction to any given circumstance? Is man no more than a product of many conditional and environmental factors...be they biological, psychological or sociological? Is man but an accidental product of these? Does man have no choice of action in the face of such circumstances?" [3]

One day, naked and alone in a small room, Frankl became acutely aware that apathy could be overcome, irritability suppressed, that he could preserve a vestige of spiritual freedom and independence of mind. The Nazis didn't have the power to take away from him his personal dignity and self-esteem unless he gave it to them. They could do what they wanted with his body, but not control the last of the human freedoms: to choose one's attitude in any given set of circumstances, to choose one's own way. Frankl recalls:

> "And there were always choices to make. Every day, every hour, offered opportunities to make a decision, a decision which determined whether you would or would not submit to those powers which threatened to rob you of your very self, your inner freedom, which determined whether or not you would become the plaything of circumstances, renouncing freedom and dignity to become molded into the form of the typical inmate...

> "In the final analysis, it becomes clear that the sort of person the prisoner became was the result of an inner decision and not the result of camp influences alone. Fundamentally, therefore, any person can, even under such circumstances, decide what shall become of him...mentally or spiritually. He may retain his dignity even in a concentration camp." [4]

Through a series of mental, emotional and moral disciplines, he became an inspiration to those around him, until even some of the prison guards began to admire him for his exhibition of dignity.

I cite this example to illustrate that even under the absolute worst of circumstances, a person is not "victim" or "captive" unless she chooses to be. If Victor Frankl could identify choices in response to his horrific dilemma, most certainly no one reading this book should feel powerless to deal with her work conflicts.

As a hospital human resource professional, I counsel employees on all levels to help them gain a greater measure of control over their work lives. At every opportunity, I share with employees how to steer clear of self-defeating behavior and instill in them a sense of responsibility for the impact their attitudes or behaviors have on others. I always view them as adults who have adult decisions to make and who must be accountable for their own actions. I never buy into an employee's perception that she is captive or victim to a problem situation, regardless of how eloquently she feigns helplessness.

Regardless of the work problem or the person experiencing it, all employees have four options from which to choose. These four options are fully described in the following chapters.

▲

Notes:

It is easier to pull down
than to build up.

Latin Proverb

▲

Chapter 6

GRIPE AND DUMP:

Option #1

As hard as you look, you will never be able to find an organization that is free of problems or conflicts. There will always be factors inherent in your job that are unpleasant, frustrating or inhibiting. You have choices in response to these problems. You can approach the situation in a constructive, collaborative manner that facilitates resolution of the difficulty or respond in a way that aggravates and escalates the problem. You can pay attention to what is good and right within the organization and take full advantage of these things, or you can dwell on the negative, obsess on everything that's wrong, causing you to display an overall negative attitude. Enter the gripe and dumper.

Most gripe and dumpers do not make a conscious choice to be overly negative, resistant to change and contrary beyond reason. There is no malicious intent. They don't wake up one morning, look in the mirror and decide, "Today, I'm going to gripe and dump, moan and groan, or whine and pout." Furthermore, the gripe and dumper is usually in the least objective position to see herself as others do. She may really believe that she is the only one in the department who cares enough, or is willing to risk enough to complain. She may feel that she is standing up for what's right or fair, and is identifying a real problem that needs looking into. She may perceive herself as the loyal "devil's advocate," making an honest attempt to improve the quality of patient care or employee relations.

Unfortunately, the gripe and dumper's *style* of addressing the problem is so abrasive and defensive-inducing, she turns people off. In fact, her style calls more attention to herself, and she can't become an effective change-agent or problem-solver because her approach gets in the way. She doesn't speak in a manner that makes others willing to listen to her. She also doesn't listen in a manner that makes others willing to talk to her. She prefers grand-standing and ego-tripping over calm dialogue. She prefers accusing and blaming people over collaborating and problem-solving.

The gripe and dumper doesn't fight fairly. She talks to everyone but the person with whom she's having a problem. She will go around the person (back biting, gossiping) or she will go over the person (tattling), instead of talking directly, honestly, and respectfully to the other person. If she does choose to confront the person, she unleashes stinging personal criticism in full public view of others, providing no face-saving for the other person.

She attacks the person rather than address the issue. She uses language that is inflammatory and divisive. She raises her voice. She interrupts. She stamps her foot. She waves her finger in the other's face. She uses negatively loaded words or phrases such as "stupid," "incompetent," "what's the matter with you" or "I thought I told you..."

The gripe and dumper never gives others the benefit of the doubt when they cross her. Instead, she always assigns malicious intent. Because she is so obsessed with who started the problem or who is to blame, she rarely takes responsibility for a problem or offers any solution that includes change on her part. She is too busy judging the motivation or behavior of others and is too overwhelmed by feelings of being victimized to be a constructive team player.

The gripe and dumper also has unrealistic expectations of the time it takes to solve a problem. She has an insatiable need for immediate gratification, and as a consequence, advances simplistic, quick-fix remedies to complex issues. Because of her inability to tolerate or adapt to everyday frustrations, she "goes to the mat" on every minor problem. In other words, she doesn't choose her fights with discretion. Every dispute, regardless of magnitude, is the hill she's willing to die on. She is like the child who too often cries "wolf," and when a real problem does arise deserving serious attention, no one takes her seriously. The manager and co-workers resign themselves to the proposition that nothing will ever make this person happy, so they stop trying. They may feign attention, but few people take this person seriously.

The gripe and dumper is also a dogmatist. She thinks that she has a corner on the truth, that her way of perceiving a problem is the only way, and that anyone who disagrees with her is either stupid or crazy. She divides co-workers into two camps: like-minded people are competent, intelligent, and morally correct. Anyone who doesn't look, think, or act like her, however, is incompetent, ignorant or morally corrupt. "You agree with me," says the gripe and dumper, "then you're my friend and we can work well together. But if you oppose me on this one, you're my enemy, which means I can't be friendly or cooperate with you until you change."

The most malicious and repugnant form of gripe and dumping, however, occurs when the person intentionally agitates, picks on, or taunts co-workers. Bored when everyone is cooperating with one another, the gripe and dumper likes to stir things up. She doesn't often engage in open mischief. She plants the seeds of discontent in private, one-on-one discussions. During department meetings, for example, she is curiously silent when given an opportunity to openly voice concerns or suggest ways to improve the working environment. As soon as the meeting adjourns, however, she engages in animated discussions, lamenting how nothing was accomplished: "Do you believe we spent an hour at that meeting? What a total waste of time. This decision will never work! Did you hear the stupid remark Jane made? Did you see the look on her face when..."

With the instincts of a guerrilla fighter, the gripe and dumper becomes a catalyst for intergroup conflict. Typical statements made by gripe and dumpers are: "They always get everything they want. Nobody cares about us. How come we always have to help them? We do our part, why can't they? We're the only ones who seem to be working around here. Do you think they're worth the money they get paid?" The gripe and dumper also thrives on division among workers in different job classifications, between shifts or departments, and in particular between employees and the manager. Nothing the manager does is ever enough for the gripe and dumper.

She resists and rejects her manager's leadership by constantly second-guessing decisions and demonstrating a serious inability to accept direction. She displays a prima donna attitude, preferring to do things her own way. She doesn't legitimize or sanction the manager's right to assign her work, counsel and evaluate her work performance, take corrective action, etc. In fact, she secretly believes that the boss is a burden and a meddler.

The gripe and dumper is usually too "street wise" to actually refuse a management directive and risk losing her job by being insubordinate. She won't say to the manager, "I'm not going to listen to you" or "Take this job and shove it." Instead, she reluctantly agrees to do what the manager asks, but then does something else. When the manager gets upset that the assignment was not completed as directed, the gripe and dumper responds in a passive–aggressive manner, relying on alibis such as: "I got busy and didn't have time to do it" (helplessness); "That's not what I heard you say" (misunderstanding); "I forgot" (memory lapse); "I tried to do what you asked, but it didn't work for me. So I did it my way" (paralysis).

The gripe and dumper is passive–aggressive toward co-workers as well as toward the manager. If she is upset with someone, she is capable of walking right past the person in the hallway without acknowledging her presence. No eye contact. No smile. No exchange of pleasantries such as, "Hello" or "How are you." In the lounge area, she offers everyone coffee, except for the person with whom she's upset. She gets up from a table and leaves if the other person sits down. She won't even let the person know why she's upset. If the person asks her to explain what's wrong, she replies, "Nothing! I don't have a problem. Do *you?*" She continues to communicate her frustration, however, in non-verbal ways. She sighs loudly. She mumbles something under her breath. She refuses to talk. She bangs the desk drawer or slams the office door shut.

When the co-worker inquires as to what's troubling her, the gripe and dumper replies, "You see, that's exactly the problem. You don't even *know* what you did!" And the pouting continues ad nauseum. When she finally decides to disclose what she's so upset about, however, an emotional outburst of pent-up aggression is unleashed. The overall tone of her remarks is one of "Shame on you. You're to blame. You started this problem. You are responsible for my behavior."

Some gripe and dumpers complain, agitate, or play the martyr role for years. Yet they refuse to quit, preferring to remain unhappy in the same job. When asked if things are going to improve within the foreseeable future, the gripe and dumper's typical response is, "No. This place will never change. Nobody really cares about us. Nobody wants to listen to our ideas." When asked why she chooses to stay if the outlook is so bleak, her response is, "I can't quit because I'll lose my seniority. I can't take a cut in pay. I'm too old to quit and learn a new job. I'm too tired to go back to school. I don't know if I could succeed doing anything else. This job, if nothing else, is secure. I can't take the risk of starting over, being last hired and first fired."

Not taking a risk, however, is sometimes a greater risk. Life is too short to spend it griping and dumping, feeling captive, victimized and powerless. Leading a life of quiet desperation is a *choice*. Gripe and dumpers choose to be unhappy because they refuse to take responsibility for their own feelings or behavior. Or they don't realize that there exist three alternative responses to job conflict that are far more constructive and self-promoting.

▲

Notes:

There is no problem so difficult it can't be solved. If it can't be solved, it's not a problem. It is a reality. We must accept realities and resolve the problems that come with them.

▲

Chapter 7

ADJUST:

Option #2

Every morning when you awake to your alarm clock, rise from bed, wash, get dressed and come to work, you have made a decision, that at least for today, the advantages outweigh the disadvantages of staying in your present job. As long as you have made this affirmative choice, it behooves you to take full advantage of all positive aspects of your job, adapt to and minimize the negative effect of those problems you can't do anything about, and make an effort to be constructive in all of your work relationships. When you choose to adjust to the imperfections in the workplace, you are following the tenets of St. Francis of Assisi when he prayed:

> "God, let me have the determination to change what I can change, the serenity to accept what I cannot, and the wisdom to know the difference between the two."

Yes, you should have the courage to deal with those work frustrations that can be reduced or eliminated. But like it or not, some things are out of your control to change, and it's better to gracefully accept reality when you cannot change it.

Successful adaptation requires maintaining realistic expectations of your co-workers and your working conditions. Try to overcome problems if, in fact, they are truly resolvable. But first diagnose the problem to determine if it is:

1. inevitable
2. an inherent condition of the work
3. outside your control to change

If the problem fits into any one of these categories, you should make an all-out attempt to adjust or accommodate yourself to the situation. After all, why continuously ram your head against a brick wall, trying to move an immovable object, when all this does is give you a headache?

As long as you continue to remain in your present position, don't view yourself as captive or victim of your situation. As a self-managed employee, you have chosen to work where you do. Economic conditions may limit your options to do something else, but for now it does little good (and much harm) to feel sorry, resent yourself and others around you, and constantly remind yourself how bad things are.

Agonizing about the job's imperfections is almost always self-defeating. You won't like yourself and you will be difficult to work with. Furthermore, your negative attitude will cause others to react defensively toward you. Your behavior influences their behavior, and you unknowingly create a negative self-fulfilling prophesy. Finally, your depression or hostility regarding things outside your ability to change will prevent you from successfully dealing with those work problems that are within your control.

Samuel Johnson observed: "The fountain of content must spring up in the mind, and he who hath so little knowledge of human nature as to seek happiness by changing anything but his own disposition, will waste his life in fruitless efforts and multiply the grief he proposes to remove."

Even though you cannot change or control all negative aspects of the working environment, you can choose not to be inordinately jostled about by these problems. You can choose to graciously and peacefully accept the problems and learn to live with them, even though you don't like them. In this way, you don't empower the problems to control you. You place them in proper perspective by taking full advantage of what's good and right within the organization and focusing on those things that are within your sphere of influence.

Successfully adapting to inherent frustrations and limitations in your work life is a mark of personal maturity. Adjusting to those job imperfections that you can't do anything about is also a survival skill. Without this ability, you are likely to take premature stands, inadvertently play the role of the martyr, and set yourself up for frustration and failure.

Identifying What Satisfies and Frustrates You on the Job

Epectetus said, "There is only one way to establish happiness and that is to cease worrying about things which are beyond the power of our will."

There exists no perfect working environment free of frustrations or irritations. As a self-managed employee, you take full advantage of the positive aspects of the job, try to change those things that are within your control to change and adjust to those things you cannot change. You always remain flexible in your dealings with customers, managers and co-workers.

Are your expectations of others realistic? Can you adjust to the job's imperfections? To determine the answer to these questions, complete the following exercises:

On the next page, list all of those things about your organization, specific job responsibilities and the people with whom you work which you truly appreciate. These are the factors that keep you coming back to work and contribute to your overall satisfaction on the job ▶

Aspects of the job that you appreciate

(Include organization, job responsibilities or people with whom you work)

▲

-
-
-
-
-
-
-
-
-
-

continued...

Identifying What Satisfies and Frustrates You on the Job

...continued

Now, make a list of those things about the job that are unpleasant. These are the factors that inhibit your job satisfaction or performance. Also determine which of these undesirable work factors are *within* or *outside* your direct control to change ▶

Frustrating
aspects of your job
(Include organization, job responsibilities or people with whom you work)

Is the problem within your control to change?

	YES	No
•	——	——
•	——	——
•	——	——
•	——	——
•	——	——
•	——	——
•	——	——
•	——	——
•	——	——
•	——	——

continued...

Review the preceding lists and objectively compare the advantages versus the disadvantages of remaining in your present job. If the advantages of staying in your position outweigh the immediate need to separate from it, then resolve to:

1. Take full advantage of the positive aspects of your job. Pay attention to what is good and right within your organization and the people with whom you work. Don't constantly knock your head against the wall reminding yourself (and others) about how bad things are, particularly if you have no control to change these things.

2. Adjust to those job frustrations that are outside your control to change and minimize their negative effect on your job satisfaction and performance. Always hold yourself responsible for doing the best you can, and remember that you are always accountable for your own behavior in response to difficult situations, regardless how others may behave.

3. If the problem is within your control to change, do what you can in a constructive manner to become part of the solution. But before you approach anyone about the issue, review the following pages to determine how (or if) you should address the problem.

▲

Notes:

Man's unique reward is that while animals survive by adjusting themselves to their background, man survives by adjusting his background to himself.

Ayn Rand

▲

Chapter 8

SEPARATE FROM JOB

Option #3

Perhaps the problems that you experience are so serious or all consuming that they cast a shadow over the positive elements of the job. Perhaps you truly cannot adjust to or tolerate the frustration. The advantages of staying simply don't outweigh the disadvantages. If this is the case, it's time to gracefully separate from your job.

Resigning from a position should be viewed as a last resort, an action to be taken only after exhausting all attempts to resolve the problem. But sometimes quitting makes the most sense, particularly if your negative attitude results in behavior that is harmful to yourself and aggravating to others.

A voluntary resignation from your job is also very practical if you find yourself on a collision course with your boss. Try to avoid at all costs getting fired. Don't place yourself in a position of losing control over your own career. Don't allow your boss to decide for you when to stay or leave. Separate from the job under your own terms and conditions when the time is right for you.

Until you find a better job, play it straight. Do what is expected of you and more. Prove to yourself, co-workers and the boss that you can rise above the differences of opinion, the personality disputes and daily irritations of the job. Demonstrate a willingness and ability to perform your tasks in an above competent manner. Don't threaten your job security by acting in a way that communicates to others: "I could care less about losing this job." In short, don't burn bridges behind you.

Consider your present job as a link in the chain or a springboard for finding a position that is more suitable to your needs. It is always easier to find a job when you have one than when you don't. Being *forced* out of your job under a cloud of suspicion and hostility will only decrease your chances of landing a more desirable position. Most companies do not look kindly at transferring a trouble-maker from one place in the organization to another. And your boss always has the power to give a bad reference, making it difficult for you to land on your feet elsewhere within a reasonable time frame.

If you have determined that sooner or later you will be separating from your present job, make every effort to temporarily adjust to the problems you face. Don't spend a great deal of energy complaining about the situation, making yourself and everyone around you miserable. Don't threaten your boss by delivering an ultimatum (however subtle) that you will quit unless your problems are immediately eliminated. She is likely to call your bluff and the smart money bets on things being resolved in the boss' favor.

▲

Job Satisfaction Audit

How do you feel about each of the following on your job? Identify your level of satisfaction by circling one number in each line across:

How satisfied are you with...

1. Your organization in comparison with other healthcare organizations you know about?

2. Your specific job tasks and responsibilites?

3. Your physical working conditions?

4. The way people in your department cooperate with one another?

5. Your supervisor's skills in managing people?

6. Your supervisor's skills in managing her own technical and administrative responsibilites?

7. Your pay, considering your duties and responsibilities?

8. Your pay, considering what other organizations pay for similar types of work?

9. The amount of recognition you receive on the job?

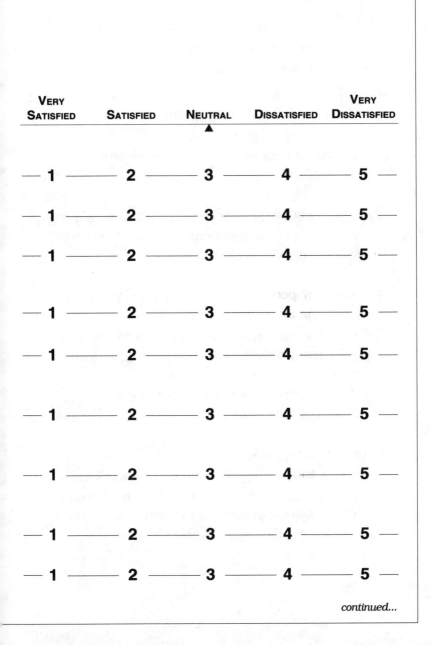

continued...

Job Satisfaction Audit

...continued

10. The extent to which your present job makes full use of your skills and abilities?

11. Opportunities for professional growth or promotion?

12. Opportunity for independent problem solving, exercise of judgment, and control over your working environment?

13. Time demands of your present job?

14. Considering everything, how would you rate your overall feelings about your employment situation at this time?

15. If you have your way, will you be working for your present organization five years from now? *(I'll be retired in five years = 0)*

VERY SATISFIED	**SATISFIED**	**NEUTRAL** ▲	**DISSATISFIED**	**VERY DISSATISFIED**

— 1 ——— 2 ——— 3 ——— 4 ——— 5 —

— 1 ——— 2 ——— 3 ——— 4 ——— 5 —

— 1 ——— 2 ——— 3 ——— 4 ——— 5 —

— 1 ——— 2 ——— 3 ——— 4 ——— 5 —

— 1 ——— 2 ——— 3 ——— 4 ——— 5 —

CERTAINLY	**PROBABLY**	**I'M NOT AT ALL SURE** ▲	**PROBABLY NOT**	**CERTAINLY NOT**

— 1 ——— 2 ——— 3 ——— 4 ——— 5 —

continued...

Job Satisfaction Audit ———

...continued

Scoring:

Add together the numbers you
circled on the Job Satisfaction
Audit and enter the total here: _____

Scores on the Audit can range between 14 and 75.
Scores of 45 or more may suggest that the overall
context of your work is less than satisfactory. You
should also evaluate the specific items in the Audit
which you rated positively or negatively.

Your rating on this questionnaire serves as a "snap-
shot" of your overall job satisfaction and can assist
you in making critical career decisions.

Notes:

Is It Time To Separate?

Examine These Questions Before You Act

Have you decided to quit in a rash moment or when emotionally upset?

                                        YES ___ NO ___

Comment:

Resignation (oral or written) is often considered an irreversible decision. Think it through before you declare your intent. You may not be able to take it back.

Are you separating when the time and conditions are convenient for you?

                                        YES ___ NO ___

Comment:

Place yourself in a position where you don't feel pressured to leave, for example, having to quit before you get fired or "beating the boss to the punch." You may need time to make your best career move, and you can buy this time by doing a competent job on your present position. Remember, it's usually easier to land a new job when you currently possess one than when you don't.

Perhaps you have already found another job and are working the last weeks in your current position. Are you inadvertently burning your bridges behind you?

YES ____   No ____

Comment:
You never know how well you like your future job until you get there. And even if you are highly successful in your new position, there may come a time when you want to return to your current organization in some other capacity. Therefore, make it your number one objective to separate with working relationships intact.

Have you exhausted all reasonable means to resolve the problem or make a satisfactory adjustment to it?

YES ____   No ____

Comment:
If you resign over every frustration or irritation that comes your way, you will get the reputation of a "job-hopper" or "unstable." Future employers look suspiciously at a job application that reflects a series of short term stints.

continued...

Is It Time To Separate?

...continued

Have you looked long and hard at the advantages versus disadvantages of accepting the new job?

Yes ___ No ___

Comment:

The grass always appears greener in the other pasture, but as you get closer to it, you begin to see the brown spots and weeds, etc. You may not have the same problems in the new job that you currently experience, but it's guaranteed that there will be another set of problems with which to cope. Second, just because another organization wants you (approval is very seductive), it doesn't necessarily mean that taking the position is the best career move. Think it through.

Notes:

Don't Shoot Yourself in the Foot

Perhaps the disadvantages of staying in your present job outweigh the advantages. It may be time to look around. If you don't think you can change things for the better and feel hopelessly frustrated, remember, no one is captive or victim to her work problems unless she chooses to be.

List below all the things
you can do in your present position
that will sabotage your ability to land a
better job within or outside your organization
▲

Let's assume it might take a little while before you can find a more suitable position. How you behave in your present job will largely determine your ability to find a better one.

***List all the things
you can do in your present job
so you can quit under your own terms,
when the time is right for you***

▲

Notes:

He has a right to criticize
who has a heart to help.

Abraham Lincoln

————— ▲ —————

Chapter 9

MANAGE THE CONFLICT:

Option #4

Successfully dealing with work problems requires effective "change-agent" skills. But before you try to address a particular conflict with your boss or co-worker, it is important to understand that you really don't have the power to control or change anyone. Control over others is an illusion. Ultimately, a person is free to behave any way she chooses, and will do so based upon her own perceived self-interests. You can provide feedback to someone, explaining how her behavior is obstructing the accomplishment of your goals. You can even request that the person change her actions in some way that will make your job more satisfying or effective. But you don't have the power to change her. You can issue demands, you can plead, cajole, nag, whine or threaten, but until she's ready to change, the behavior will continue.

It is also important to understand that you are not responsible or accountable for another person's behavior. You are always responsible for your own actions, however, and because you have direct control over this area, it is the best place to begin your change efforts. In fact, sometimes your best hope for establishing a positive relationship with a difficult boss or co-worker is to be introspective regarding your own behavior and its effect on the other person. When you demonstrate a willingness to first change yourself, you make it easier for the other person to change in the direction you desire. The following exercise will help you focus on your own areas of control as you attempt to successfully manage a job conflict.

A Self-Management Exercise to Resolve Co-Worker Conflict

The advantage of this conflict-resolution procedure is that it doesn't require direct involvement of your boss or consent of the co-worker. You can do it on your own even without the other person knowing it. It is advantageous, of course, for the boss or co-worker to be a willing partner in the exercise, but this is not necessary to achieve positive results. In fact, your ability to take independent action, regardless of the other's inclination to do likewise, is the value of this exercise.

Step 1:
Develop a List of the Boss or Co-Worker's Good Qualities

Recognize and acknowledge what she is doing right. What behaviors do you observe in her that you appreciate and wish to continue? Unfortunately, when a working relationship has gone sour, you have a tendency to overlook (or take for granted) these positive qualities in a person. But, you run the risk of extinguishing those behaviors you appreciate in a person when you choose to ignore them. Good behavior needs reinforcement. The person needs to know that you notice when she's doing things to make your job easier, more satisfying, or more effective. Therefore, the first step in resolving the conflict is to develop a laundry list of what the boss or co-worker is doing right.

Step 2:
List Your Bad Habits

Consider what you have done in the past to provoke the other person. Recall her complaints or requests for change on your part. Then develop a laundry list of what you do too much or too little of that probably frustrates your boss or co-worker. If you're not certain how to complete this list, place yourself in the other person's shoes. What would she say you do too much or too little of that frustrates her? It doesn't matter whether the person is right or wrong or whether you do these things intentionally. If she might perceive that you do too much or too little of something, include it in this list.

Step 3:
Develop Commitments For Behavioral Change

Review your list of bad habits (as perceived by your boss or co-worker) and determine which behaviors you are willing to change to improve the working relationship. Write down three things that you're going to do more or less of that will increase your chances for cooperation with the person. Be certain that you commit to things that you are *willing* and *able* to accomplish within a reasonable time-frame. Also, make certain that your three commitments for change will be observable to the boss or co-worker. It's not enough to state, for example, that "I will improve my attitude" or that "I will take more initiative to help you." What will you do specifically to improve your attitude or to demonstrate greater initiative? In other words, describe your commitments in behavioral terms.

Step 4:
Initiate A Meeting With the Boss or Co-Worker

After you have completed the previous steps, initiate a confidential meeting with the person to explain the thought processes you've gone through and share your information. It is entirely possible that the person will be just a little bit stunned and suspicious of this whole process. Anticipate and plan for potential resistance, and be determined that regardless of the other's response, you will remain positive. Don't get upset or give up even if the person demonstrates a defensive posture throughout the duration of the meeting. Remember, your boss or co-worker cannot make you act defensively or hostile. You are responsible for your own behavior.

Continuously ask for feedback from the person as you share the information contained in your three lists. Solicit her ideas, check for clear communication, and align yourself with her thoughts. It is particularly important for you not to get angry if she readily agrees with everything you mentioned on your second list (those things you do that bother her). Her agreement simply shows that you were successful in seeing the world through her eyes.

When you divulge your list of commitments, ask the person to accept these behavioral changes as good faith gestures to improve the working relationship. If necessary, be prepared to develop new commitments based upon the person's feedback. State that you intend to act immediately on these behavioral change commitments, and request that she give you constructive feedback when she observes you are not living up to them.

Your efforts will be wasted if you do not deliver on your commitments to improve the working relationship. Even if the co-worker does not choose to offer commitments of her own to improve the relationship, you have accomplished three things by engaging in this exercise:

1. You have become more introspective regarding your behavior and its effect upon the person.

2. You have made it easier for the person to change by demonstrating a willingness to first change yourself.

3. You have done your part to break the deadlock by acting responsibly. The ball is now in your boss or co-worker's court to respond in kind.

Confronting a Co-Worker's Negative Behavior

When it becomes necessary to confront a co-worker to address actions that have a negative impact on your job, it is important to check your intentions. If your *real* goal is to threaten, punish, seek revenge, insult, berate, justify and defend your position, or dictate the resolution of the conflict, then there exists little chance of gaining voluntary compliance to your wishes. This approach has a clear "me versus you" orientation. Your energy is directed toward total victory or dominance. You are articulating the problem strictly from your own point of view, rather than defining the issue in terms of mutual needs. The conflict is likely to get personal and ugly. This aggressive approach might serve as a nice catharsis for you, but it will only create defensiveness and polarization, and result in a breakdown of communication and cooperation between you and the other person.

If aggression doesn't work, neither does passivity. A passive person denies or smooths over real problems, avoids any situation that is conflict-prone, agrees with the other person (when she really doesn't), takes the blame when she doesn't deserve it, and gossips to third parties. The passive person often resents herself for her self-imposed powerlessness, and she displaces her frustrations onto others who are not directly involved in the conflict. The passive approach is dysfunctional because it prevents any opportunity for meaningful dialogue and resolution of the conflict. Successful conflict management requires the willingness to talk directly, honestly and respectfully with others. It requires assertive confrontation and the ability to fight fairly.

———————▲———————

Conduct a Realistic Analysis of Your Work Problems

Can the problem really be solved?

Yᴇs ___   No ___

Comment:

If the situation is outside your control to change, your objective should be to:

1. adjust to the problem and minimize its negative impact on you, or
2. separate from the situation with your self-respect intact. Griping and dumping will only make you and others miserable.

Is the problem so serious that you can't adjust to it?

Yᴇs ___   No ___

Comment:

If you complain about every minor job inconvenience or irritation and always want to have things your way, you will be viewed as a gripe and dumper. When a really serious problem *does* come up, no one will take you seriously. Remember the lad who called "wolf" too often...

**Will the problem go away by itself if
you do nothing?**

YES ___ **No** ___

Comment:
Sometimes "doing less is more". Some problems simply have a way of correcting themselves without you having to do anything. In fact, your reactions could be making the situation worse.

Even if you didn't start the problem, have you honestly examined your behavior to determine if you're aggravating the situation in some way?

YES ___ **No** ___

Comment:
Remember, you are always responsible for your own actions, regardless of how others may behave.

continued...

Conduct a Realistic Analysis of Your Work Problems

...continued

Is it really your problem?

YES ___ **No** ___

Comment:
Don't fight someone else's battle or get sucked into a conflict when it is not really your concern. Life is too short to be constantly embroiled in unnecessary conflict.

Are you talking directly with the person who is upsetting you?

YES ___ **No** ___

Comment:
Sometimes we talk to everyone *but* the person who is the source of the conflict. Back-stabbing and undermining is almost always self-defeating.

Have you asked for help to solve the problem?

YES ___ **No** ___

Comment:
Perhaps someone in your organization is in an objective position to give you feedback on how to handle the situation. This person may also be in a position to help you mediate the conflict or offer other resources.

Are you looking for a quick fix solution?

YES ___ NO ___

Comment:
If you try to change things too quickly, you can make the situation worse. Always try to assess the readiness of people to change.

Is the issue worth losing a relationship over?

YES ___ NO ___

Comment:
Sometimes it is wise to compromise or give in when the issue is of greater importance to the other person, or when continuous fighting will only further harm the relationship.

What's your chance of winning if you go "toe-to-toe" with the other person?

YES ___ NO ___

Comment:
Don't set yourself up for defeat or play the martyr role unless this is "the hill you're willing to die on."

Establishing Effective Work Relationships

Whether or not you personally like a co-worker, boss, or customer, maintaining a good working relationship will make your job easier, more satisfying and effective. Good working relationships, in fact, grease the results channels for you to survive and thrive on the job.

A. List below specific attitudes or behaviors that should be displayed toward *co-workers* (whether or not you like them on a personal level) to demonstrate your on-the-job maturity and professionalism:

B. List below specific attitudes or behaviors that should be displayed toward your *boss* and other *"higher-up's"* in the organization that will maximize your chances for job success and satisfaction:

C. List below specific attitudes or behaviors that should be displayed toward *customers*, particularly when they have a challenging question or complaint:

D. List below specific attitudes or behaviors that should be displayed toward your *organization*, despite your feelings at times regarding its quality of decisions or style of individual management:

Technical Skills Are Not Enough

Technically competent employees sometimes place their jobs in jeopardy because of an inability to:

- Adjust to frustrations of the job or deal constructively with work problems.

- Establish an effective relationship with the boss or other influential people within the organization.

- Successfully manage conflicts with co-workers.

- Successfully manage demanding or challenging customers.

On the following page, give an example of someone, who despite her technical skills, placed her job in jeopardy. Discuss the nature of the conflict and list: (1) specific "gripe and dump" behaviors exhibited by the individual that were observable to boss, co-workers, or customers, and (2) specific attitudes or behaviors the individual *could* have exhibited that may have achieved a better outcome ▶

***Specific "gripe and dump" behaviors that were
observable to boss, co-workers, or customers***
▲

***Specific attitudes or behaviors
that may have achieved a better outcome***
▲

Notes:

You cannot shake hands
with a clenched fist.

Indira Gandhi

▲

Chapter 10

FAIR-FIGHTING TECHNIQUES

Assertiveness is a collaborative approach to conflict geared toward a "win-win" outcome. When you are assertive, you attempt to de-personalize the conflict; that is, you channel your energies toward solving the problem rather than defeating the other person. You make a real attempt to *understand* the feelings of the other person as opposed to *judging* the other person. As a result, both of you can have your needs met.

When you are assertive, you simply describe the problem from your point of view and the negative effect this problem is having on you. You communicate the problem without attacking the person and you remain constructive regardless of how the other person chooses to behave.

Listed in this chapter are specific assertive, fair-fighting strategies which will increase your chances for effectively managing on-the-job conflicts.

1. *Don't expect perfection in others.* Try to maximize people's strengths, minimize their weaknesses and adjust to their imperfections. If you expect perfection in others, you are destined to lead a life of self-righteous, ulcerous indignation. If you expect perfection in yourself, you are destined to lead a life of guilt and frustration.

2. *Choose your fights with discretion.* Some problems aren't worth complaining about. If you gripe about every little thing, you will gain the reputation of "complainer" or "agitator." Furthermore, nobody will take you seriously when a real problem does require someone's attention.

3. *Talk directly to the person with whom you're having the problem.* Sometimes, employees talk to everyone but the person with whom they're having the problem. This creates a breakdown of communication and distrust.

4. *Talk to the person behind closed doors* within the spirit of confidentiality and non-competitiveness. Don't criticize anyone in public. It only leads to embarrassment and raises a person's defensiveness.

5. *Be cool, calm and collected* when you confront the person with a problem. Don't lead with your emotions; avoid yelling, swearing, interrupting, crying. Don't wave the finger of blame, shame and guilt. Be mindful of the effect that your message (verbal and non-verbal) will have on the other person. Your

feedback should make it easier, not harder, for the person to change in the desired direction.

6. *Be issue-oriented,* not personality-oriented. Simply describe the person's behavior (without attacking her) and the negative effects this behavior has on you.

7. *Be open to different interpretations of the same event.* After all, you don't have a corner on the truth. You only have your perceptions of reality. Share your point of view with the person and ask for hers.

8. *Don't sandbag or collect misdeeds,* thereby building up personal resentment for the person. Deal with one issue at a time as they arise. The best feedback is usually immediate feedback as long as you have control over how you're going to approach the person.

9. *Discretion is the better part of valor* and brutal honesty is not always a virtue. Don't say anything to the person that you will later regret. Don't unleash your severest blow. Once you say something in anger, you cannot take it back. The person may forgive you, but may never forget what you said.

10. *Give everyone you deal with an opportunity to save face and keep self-esteem intact.* This is particularly important when you know that you are right on an issue. Give the person "wiggle room" to maneuver rather than backing her into a corner and inviting unnecessary defensiveness.

11. *Know when to terminate the discussion.* If, in the course of a confrontation, you (or the other person) have repeated your best arguments more than once, it is likely that you're "beating a dead horse" or going around in circles. Agree to disagree for the time being and come back to the discussion later if necessary.

12. *Get a third party resource* when appropriate to help mediate the conflict. Sometimes you need to talk with someone who has psychological and objective distance to give you advice on how to handle the conflict.

13. *Know when to put the conflict behind you* and "start a new day." Not all work conflicts can be resolved, but as a professional you have to manage these conflicts in an effective manner. Don't get stuck in a conflict mode. There will always be conflicts in a close relationship, but in between the conflicts try to reaffirm the positive aspects of working together.

14. *Don't use personal dislikes as an excuse for a poor working relationship.* Remember, you don't need to like someone on a personal basis in order to work effectively with her. Liking someone is not a precondition for a successful working relationship. Whether you like someone or not, effective communication and cooperation are expected and necessary if you are to be successful in your job.

15. *Don't violate any of the above fair-fighting principles* even if the other person chooses to ignore them. You are always accountable for your own behavior regardless of provocation.

The *Aikido* Method of Self-Defense: A Strategy for Assertive Confrontation

In the Western culture, we are conditioned to respond to force (physical or verbal) by applying equal or greater force in order to win, overcome, control or subdue. This strategy often leads to greater resistance from the aggressor, resulting in a battle over who has greater strength or will power.

In the *Aikido* method of self-defense, you don't automatically go toe-to-toe with your opponent. You don't frontally resist or get in her way. Rather, you use the person's own force or forward momentum against herself. As the *Aikido* master anticipates the moment of physical contact, her competitive advantage is her sense of balance and inward control over her physical and mental processes. She is extremely observant of her opponent's every move. She stays within herself. Instead of directly resisting the force, the *Aikido* master steps aside, deflects the person's energy, gets a hold of the opponent, and brings her down in the same direction she was going. The pivotal point in the conflict occurs when the opponent expects resistance and doesn't get it.

The *Aikido* method of self-defense works equally well with verbal assaults, when you are dealing with an angry or demanding person. The following six-step process is designed to deflect a person's negative energy rather than resist it. The purpose is to establish a win-win rather than a win-lose outcome.

Step #1:
Understand Where the Individual Is Coming From

When a person is upset and demanding, her most fundamental need is to be *understood*, not necessarily agreed with. Therefore, if you want to calm her down and get her to be more reasonable, the first strategy is to actively listen to her. Listen to her as if it is the first time you ever heard this problem. At various times during this process, insert remarks such as "I understand," "Yes," and "Go on." Use non-verbal gestures that communicate your understanding of what she's saying. Be certain that you let the person exhaust all of her concerns before you reply.

Step #2:
Summarize

Paraphrase what you think you heard the person say to ensure that you got it right. An example of this is, "Let me be sure I completely understand what you said before I respond." Check for accuracy by asking, "Is that it?" "Did I accurately describe your concern?" If the answer indicates that you captured only part but not all of her concerns correctly, ask for clarification and try again to summarize to the person's satisfaction. Don't go to the next step until you get confirmation that you completely understand her position.

Step #3:
Empathize

You may strongly disagree with what the person is saying, but before you engage in a rebuttal, try to communicate an appreciation for the person's point of view. You can accomplish this in the following ways:

- Look at the world from her perspective, what she has gone through and is presently experiencing.

- Demonstrate an appreciation that her perceptions (right or wrong) are real and legitimate. You must deal with her perceptions as reality.

- Sense the person's anger, suspicion, confusion or feelings of being treated unfairly as if these were your own.

- Ask direct, open-ended questions that will enable you to define the specifics of the problem from her world view.

- Be yourself, without a front or facade, ensuring that your relationship with the person is genuine and sincere.

- Be non-judgmental. You can't empathize with a person and judge her at the same time. Empathy requires an open and non-critical perspective of the other person's point of view.

Step #4:
Clarify

- Clarify your role in helping solve the problem. Ask the person what she would like you to do to help remedy the situation (if it is not already explicitly stated). The person may only want someone to listen to her and nothing more; she may not know what you can do to solve the problem; or she may ask you to do something specifically to meet her needs.

- Determine your ability to accommodate the person. Negotiate if necessary by exploring various options. Explain your constraints and limitations. Don't refuse to do something because "It's policy." Try to explain the *reasons* for the policy. Ask yourself if it is appropriate given the situation to relax a policy to meet her specific expectations.

- Whenever possible, try to meet at least one or more of the person's needs, even if your offer is not what she originally requested. And remember, if you do offer to satisfy one of her needs, do so willingly and enthusiastically, not begrudgingly.

Step #5:
Bring In A Third Party If...

- You feel you don't have the power to satisfy the person's request, and someone else is in a better position to help.

- You feel yourself getting personally defensive and are about to "lose it."

Step #6:
Honor Commitments, Do As Promised

Follow through with your commitments, and request feedback from the person at a later time to ensure the situation has improved.

Empathy:
The Key to Effective Conflict Management

Your ability to empathize with people under stressful and strained conditions is critical if you want to successfully manage a conflict. Empathy is more than "walking in the other person's shoes" to see the world from her perspective. If you are a good empathizer, you know a person well enough to accurately predict the responses you will evoke in her based upon your approach. You will feel more secure in the working relationship because you can accurately interpret her attitudes or intentions, perceive situations from her viewpoint and anticipate her behavior in various situations. It is this ability to accurately predict her responses that enables you to avoid unnecessary friction. When disagreements do arise, the use of empathy will help you avoid inadvertent escalation of the conflict.

When you empathize, you:

1. Suspend your judgment of the co-worker just long enough to see the world through her eyes.

2. Sense the co-worker's confusion, timidity, suspicion, anger, or feelings of being treated unfairly, as if they were your own.

3. Appreciate that no matter how unreasonable, irrational or immoral the co-worker's behavior may appear to you, it is quite reasonable, rational and moral to the co-worker.

4. Reflect upon how the co-worker has responded to past behaviors on your part.

5. Predict how she might act in the future based upon what you might say or do.

6. Choose to act in a manner that you think will evoke the most positive responses in the co-worker.

Empathy requires a non-defensive, non-judgmental approach to handling differences of opinion. You cannot criticize someone and empathize with her at the same time. These are psychologically opposing states. Empathy is also very strategic. By seeing the world from the other person's point of view, it helps you anticipate and plan for resistance to your ideas. It gives you an opportunity to "package" your ideas in a manner that will be more accepting to her without compromising your basic principles. Besides, you can't completely understand your own position until you fully understand the rationale of your adversary's position. Understanding the other's point of view helps you clarify how or why you have arrived at your position in the first place.

Only secure people are willing and able to empathize. When you empathize, you take the risk of having your perspective changed. You might learn something from the psychological engagement that will alter your thinking. You may not be the same person. Insecure people are unwilling to take this chance. There is safety in certainty, and it is all too easy to dismiss ideas that run contrary to one's belief systems.

We all like to think of ourselves as intelligent, right-thinking and decent, and it is natural to build up psychological defense mechanisms to protect us from an onslaught of opposing ideas. To personally and professionally develop, however, we must be open to other perspectives and risk being transformed. Empathic people take this risk. They recognize that perception is nine-tenths of reality when it comes to interpersonal conflict, and that there is no harm in understanding, if not appreciating, a different point of view. Empathy, after all, is not agreement. It is simply acknowledging that no matter how illogical the other person's perspective is to you, it makes a great deal of sense to her given her set of experiences.

People don't necessarily "see" events the same way. When you are in conflict, therefore, it is helpful to look at things from the other's perspective. Through empathy, you may discover a creative way to resolve or manage the conflict.

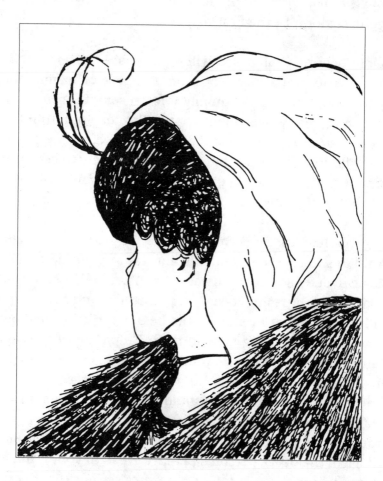

Can you see in this picture both the young and elderly woman?[5] It may require an adjustment of *perception* on your part.

Notes:

Practicing Empathy

The secret to successfully managing job conflicts is to demonstrate a willingness to understand the other person's point of view and exhibit positive behavior that demonstrates this understanding. The empathy approach makes it easier for the person to be more sensitive to your needs.

Are you in conflict with someone at work? Instead of defending your position, such as stating why you think you are right and the other person is wrong, describe the situation *from the other's point of view.* Where is this person coming from? What are this person's specific needs? Can you say or do anything differently to deal with her concerns and thus make it easier for this person to change in a positive direction?

List person's fundamental needs or expectations of you

Are you consistently meeting these needs?

▲

	Yes	No
•	——	——
•	——	——
•	——	——
•	——	——
•	——	——
•	——	——
•	——	——
•	——	——
•	——	——
•	——	——
•	——	——

continued...

Practicing Empathy

...continued

List below specific action steps you can take to better meet this individual's needs. Be specific and behaviorally concise. The actions you take should be *observable* to the other person.

Things I can *start* doing

▲

Things I can *stop* doing

▲

Lessons from *Tao* on Conflict Management

Excerpts from Lao Tzu's *Tao Te Ching* [6]

- When a person wants to fight with you, consider the strategy of the guerilla commander.

  Never seek a fight. If it comes to you, yield, step back. It is far better to step back than to overstep yourself.

  Your strength is good intelligence: be aware of what is happening.

  Advance only where you encounter no resistance. If you make a point, do not cling to it. If you win, be gracious.

  The person who initiates the attack is off-center and easily thrown. Even so, have respect for any attacker. Never surrender your compassion or use your skill to harm another needlessly.

  In any event, the more conscious force will win.

● When you are puzzled by what you see or hear, do not strive to figure things out. Stand back for a moment and become calm. When a person is calm, complex events appear simple.

To know what is happening, push less, open out and be aware. See without staring. Listen quietly rather than listening hard. Use intuition and reflection rather than trying to figure things out.

The more you can let go of trying, and the more open and receptive you become, the more easily you will know what is happening.

Also, stay in the present. The present is more available than either memories of the past or fantasies of the future.

So attend to what is happening now.

continued...

Lessons from *Tao* on Conflict Management

...continued

- Gentle interventions, if they are clear, overcome rigid resistances.

  If gentleness fails, try yielding or stepping back altogether. When the person yields, resistances relax.

- Generally speaking, a person's consciousness sheds more light on what is happening than any number of interventions or explanations.

- Being open and attentive is more effective than being judgmental. This is because people naturally tend to be good and truthful when they are being received in a good and truthful manner.

- If you are attacked or criticized, react in a way that will shed light on the event. This is a matter of being centered and of knowing that an encounter is a dance and not a threat to your ego or existence. Tell the truth.

If you are conscious of what is happening, you will recognize emerging situations long before they have gotten out of hand. Every situation, no matter how vast or complex it may become, begins both small and simple.

Neither avoid nor seek encounters, but be open and when an encounter arises, respond to it while it is still manageable. There is no virtue in delaying until heroic action is needed to set things right. In this way, potentially difficult situations become simple.

- The greatest martial arts are the gentlest. They allow an attacker the opportunity to fall down.

- The greatest generals do not rush into every battle.

continued...

Lessons from *Tao* on Conflict Management

...continued

- The wise person knows that yielding overcomes resistances, and gentleness melts rigid defenses.

  The person does not fight the force of the other's energy, but flows and yields and absorbs and lets go. This is another paradox: what is soft is strong.

- Even if harsh interventions succeed brilliantly, there is no cause for celebration. There has been injury. Someone's process has been violated.

  Later on, the person whose process has been violated may well become less open and more defended. There will be a deeper resistance and possibly even resentment.

  Making people do what you think they ought to do does not lead toward clarity and consciousness. While they may do what you tell them to do at the time, they will cringe inwardly, grow confused, and plot revenge.

  This is why your victory is actually a failure.

• To know how other people behave takes intelligence, but to know myself takes wisdom.

To manage other people's lives takes strength, but to manage my own life takes true power.

Discriminating Between Assertive, Aggressive and Passive Behavior

What Is Responsible, Assertive Behavior?

It consists of standing up for your personal rights and expressing thoughts, feelings and beliefs in direct, honest and appropriate ways which do not violate another's personal rights.

Assertive behavior is more than just saying the right words. In assertive behavior:

1. The nonverbal behaviors are congruent with the verbal messages; they add support, strength and emphasis to what is said.

2. The voice is appropriately loud for the situation.

3. Eye contact is firm, but not a stare-down.

4. Body gestures denote strength not aggression.

5. The speech pattern is fluent, without awkward hesitation; it is expressive, clear and emphasizes key words.

How Does Assertive Behavior Differ From Aggressive Behavior?

Aggressive behavior is obtaining what one wants by violating the other's personal rights. Aggressive behavior is also more than the mere statement of words. In aggressive behavior:

1. The nonverbal behaviors used are ones which dominate or demean the other person.

2. Eye contact attempts to stare-down and intimidate the other.

3. A hard and loud voice, which does not fit the situation, may be used.

4. A sarcastic or condescending tone of voice can exist.

5. "Parental" body gestures, such as excessive finger-pointing, sometimes occur.

continued...

Discriminating Between Assertive, Aggressive and Passive Behavior

...continued

How Does Passive Behavior Differ From Assertive or Aggressive Behavior?

Acting *passively* results in pacifying others and avoiding conflict at any cost. By this type of action a person violates her own personal rights by failing to express honest feelings, thoughts and beliefs. It can also be demonstrated by expressing one's thoughts and feelings in such an apologetic, timid and degrading manner that others can easily disregard them. In passive behavior, the nonverbal behaviors include:

1. Evasive eye contact.

2. Body gestures such as hand-wringing, stepping back from the other person as a strong remark is made, hunching the shoulders, stiff body posture and distracting nervous gestures.

3. A voice tone which is overly soft.

4. A speech pattern that is hesitant and filled with pauses; the throat may be cleared frequently.

5. Distracting facial gestures, such as raising of the eyebrow, laughing and winking when expressing anger.

In general, passive nonverbals are ones which convey weakness, anxiety, pleading or degradation. They reduce the impact of what is being verbalized, which is why passive people use them.

Notes:

Gentleness springs from
great strength.

R. E. Phillips

▲

Chapter 11

THE NURSE AND
THE VERBALLY ABUSIVE PHYSICIAN

A Study in Confrontation

Recently, I conducted a Conflict-Management Workshop for a group of thirty nurses and had just completed a talk on effective fair-fighting, when a participant expressed some doubts regarding the presentation. She said that she wasn't sure the confrontation techniques would be effective for dealing with a particular physician who was well-known for his obnoxious and verbally abusive communications with hospital employees. To reinforce her position, she shared with me this alarming story:

"I was sitting down at the nursing station completing a patient chart. You must understand that this is a very public place. All around me are employees within and outside my department, engaged in a variety of activities, and I am also in full view of many patients and visitors. All of a sudden when I least expect it, 'Dr. Grouch' approaches me and starts yelling at the top of his voice: 'You stupid idiot! Who in the hell do you think you are playing doctor, telling my patient that it's O.K. to get out of bed without checking this out with me first. This is irresponsible, and as far as I'm concerned it shows your total incompetence to take care of my patients. If I had anything to do with it, I'd kick your ass right out of here.' He went on like this, hovering over me, talking down to me as if I were a child in need of a lecture, waving his finger in my face, stomping his feet, acting like a tyrant with a temper tantrum."

"What did you do?" I asked. She continued,

"Well, I didn't know what to do. I was caught off guard and stunned that this could be happening to me. I felt embarrassed and humiliated. I was also extremely self-conscious, feeling as if everyone was staring at me waiting to see what I would do. I felt the tears welling up inside of me. I wanted to respond to his accusations, but every time I tried to utter a sound, he interrupted me. I remember thinking to myself that this is so unfair that I should be expected to accept this kind of treatment from a physician. I felt like standing up and telling him what he could do with his opinions, but I didn't want to get into trouble with administration. So I felt immobilized."

"How did you respond?" I asked.

"Well, I couldn't take it any more. I thought I was going to lose it and say something to him that I would later regret. So I felt the best thing I could do under the circumstances was to get up and walk away from him."

"What did he do?" I asked.

"This made him really crazy. He yelled at the top of his voice: 'Young lady, where do you think you're going. I'm not through talking with you. Don't walk away from me. Get back here right now. Do you hear me?!?'"

"What did you do then?" I asked.

"Well, at this point the tears were really rolling down my cheeks and I was visibly shaken. I didn't want to give him the satisfaction of letting him know he got to me. I just needed to get away from the situation to catch my breath. So I darted through the double doors of our medical surgical unit onto another floor to escape further confrontation."

"What did he do?" I asked.

"He *followed* me! I could hear him stomping and storming behind me yelling at the top of his lungs, 'Young lady, you can run, but you can't hide. You're going to have to talk with me sooner or later! Get back here!' Of course, now a scene was being created on another floor with people turning their heads wondering what's going on here.

As I'm scurrying down the hallway trying to get distance between us, I see out of the corner of my eye a walk-in closet door to my left that was ajar. Without another thought, I quickly darted into the closet, shut the door, held the door knob tightly, and remained there in the total dark until I was confident that he had given up and left. When I felt it was safe, I cautiously cracked open the door, looked in both directions to ensure that the coast was clear, ran out of the hospital and went home."

A kind of eerie silence fell over the group. It was a disgusting and depressing story. Before I could say anything, another nurse, clearly angry about what she had just heard, blurted out:

"Dammit! Who does he think he is treating us like that. We don't have to take this. If he ever tried that with me, it would be his last time. I'd set him back on his heels. Let him get a taste of his own medicine. Let him know how it feels to be talked at that way. Two can play this game!"

"Wait a minute," I said. "What we have here is an ugly incident provoked by an unprofessional physician. What he did is an assault to our sensibilities. But the only two responses available to the nurse that I've heard thus far are *flight* (walk away to avoid confrontation) or *fight* (resort to the same tactics as the physician). Fight and flight are the only choices available to animals when caught in the throes of a conflict: Upon sizing up the situation, if an animal instinctively knows it can't win, it runs away to save its hide. If, on the other hand, the animal believes it can overcome the threat, it will counter attack.

"Fortunately, human beings have a third, more creative choice in response to conflict. We can be *assertive*. Assertiveness, however, is not a knee-jerk reaction to a provocative situation. Assertiveness means that you have the choice to respond in a constructive manner, even if the other person is acting irresponsibly. This abusive physician does not have the power over you to dictate how you will respond. Therefore, this doctor can't force you to run away, any more than he can cause you to fly off the handle."

At this time, I shared with the group how B. F. Skinner, through experiments in classical conditioning, proved that he could accurately predict an animal's behavioral response to certain stimuli. By carefully allocating the rewards and consequences that accompany a particular stimulus, he showed that an animal would respond in a predictable fashion. Therefore, *stimulus directly causes response* in laboratory animals.

B. F. Skinner's Classical Conditioning Model

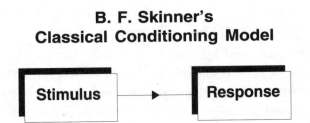

But when dealing with fully functioning human adults, the classical conditioning model for explaining behavior doesn't work. In people, there is an important gap between stimulus and response, and this gap comprises independent will and the freedom of choice. You can decide for yourself how a stimulus is going to affect you. Difficult people and provocative situations will automatically evoke certain emotions in you, like frustration or hurt. But you always have an independent choice as to how you are going to manage these feelings and act on them.[7]

Individual Responsibility Model

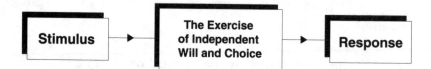

Your independent will and the freedom to choose are what make you unique. You create the meanings. You make sense of the events. You respond to various situations based upon your interpretation of the situation. You have independent will, the choice to act affirmatively and constructively regardless of how someone else is behaving. You have the choice to take responsibility for your actions and to view yourself as an independent agent.

You also have a conscience, a deep inner awareness of right versus wrong, good versus bad, moral versus immoral. If you are grounded by a set of fundamental values and are, regardless of circumstances, ethical in your dealings with people, you are less likely to falter or be compromised when a difficult choice presents itself.

You have your professionalism to consider as well, that is a sense of pride regarding your role and its importance in the organization. You are not just representing yourself on the job. You are representing all those who came before you and you are setting the stage for those who will follow you. You have a responsibility, therefore, to present your profession in the best light possible.

Finally, you have self-esteem, the value or worth you place in yourself. If you feel good about yourself and about what you're doing, you are less likely to be shaken by every criticism or disparaging remark. With self-esteem intact, you are able to respond constructively in conflict even when those around you are behaving destructively. Leo Rosten taught, "It is the weak who are cruel. Softness can only be expected from the strong." He was not speaking of physical strength but an internal resolve to believe in oneself, one's capabilities and potential for goodness.

Let's now return to the nurse's story. In the example given, the tyrannical physician did not cause the nurse to walk away. Her choice to escape was largely driven by her internal dialogue or self-talk in the midst of the assault. Her response was, in fact, a direct result of the meaning she placed in the event. As the physician was stamping his feet, yelling at the top of his voice, and speaking in a condescending tone, the nurse was saying to herself:

"This shouldn't be happening to me. This is so unfair. This is so embarrassing. Everyone must be staring at me. I feel I'm about to lose it (cry or yell). I really can't trust what I'm about to say next. I need time to think. I need to get away from this situation now."

Given this internal dialogue, it is quite natural for the nurse to flee the scene. But it was the self-talk and not the doctor that caused her response. The nurse did have a choice to interpret the event differently. As the doctor was engaged in his tirade, exhibiting his aberrant behavior, she *could* have been saying to herself:

"This man is temporarily insane! But why should I react in kind? He's not embarrassing me. He's embarrassing himself. Besides, there's no point getting personally defensive here. He does this to all the nurses. I can rise above this. Now is a great chance to display my professionalism in the face of his unprofessionalism. I'm going to handle this situation with finesse."

If the nurse had engaged in this positive self-talk instead of feeling victimized and powerless, her response would have been different. One assertive response could have been:

"Doctor, I'm as concerned about the patient as you are, and I really do want to discuss this case with you, but not *this way* and not *here* at the nursing station. Let's walk over to the conference room down the hall."

There are no guarantees. The physician might reply, "You're not telling me where to go or how I'm going to talk to you!"

The nurse could then respond:

> "Doctor, I want to get to the bottom of your complaint. But I will not stand here and be subjected to this kind of language. I believe this discussion is inappropriate, and unless we can talk about the case in a different manner, I'm going to have to leave. Now, would you like to join me in the conference room. If not, we'll have to terminate the discussion right now."

Of course, it takes a nurse with high self-esteem and confidence to respond this way under such stressful circumstances. It also takes preparation. But you can anticipate and plan for such occasions in advance of their occurring, and you can mentally practice your response. After all, this doctor has established a pattern of verbal abuse. He is predictable.

If you say to yourself, "I could never be so cool or calm under pressure like that," you are creating a negative self-fulfilling prophecy that will inhibit any opportunity for growth. A more self-promoting thought would be, "In the past, I have never had it in me to stand up to bullies, but with practice, I can get better."

On the other hand, you might say to yourself, "Assertiveness sounds good in theory. But if a physician (or anyone else) were to verbally assault me that way, I'd have no choice but to give him a taste of his own medicine." This too is a self-fulfilling prophecy. The *thought* is the problem. If you really believe that your behavior is caused by something "out there," by an external stimulus over which you have no control, that there's nothing you can do about it, then you abdicate responsibility. You are reacting to the situation instead of acting on the basis of wise choices.

Epilogue to Physician–Nurse Story

In the Conflict-Management Workshops conducted for all staff nurses within this hospital, participants practiced responding to various conflictual situations they encounter with patients, visitors, co-workers and managers. They discussed the advantages and disadvantages of different strategies and reached consensus as to the most effective assertive response to each situation. Participants were also assured by hospital management that they would be fully supported if the time came that these assertive responses would have to be utilized.

Several weeks later, I received feedback from the Vice President of Patient Care Services that nurses were consistently using their newly acquired skills as needed. And, as a result of the assertive response he was receiving from nurses, the verbally abusive physician was showing concrete evidence of positive behavior change. The Vice President also said that she had heard from her counterpart at another hospital where the physician had privileges, that he continued to be abusive with nurses at that site. But she was grateful that he had "mellowed out" dramatically in his relationship to her nurses.

This story is instructive in two ways. First, if you accept verbal abuse from certain physicians, you are, in effect, reinforcing verbal abuse. What you *accept* is what you *teach.* At some point you have to set limits of conduct and abide by them. The example is instructive in another way. The challenge of improving the physician-nurse relationship has to be accepted on an individual level. A difficult physician is more likely to be abusive with a passive nurse than he is with an assertive one. The key to effective conflict management, therefore, is to learn constructive assertiveness skills and utilize them even if someone else does not.

▲

Notes:

Let him who would move the
world first move himself.

Socrates

———————▲———————

Chapter 12

UNDERSTANDING YOUR
INNER DIALOGUE

For some people, the term "responsibility" is a negatively-charged concept associated with feelings of "should" or "guilt." But being responsible simply means holding yourself accountable for the results of your decisions or being capable of making moral and rational decisions on your own.

Taking responsibility means that you acknowledge what you bring or contribute to a conflict situation (your input), and that you have an influence on how the situation will be resolved. You can assess your specific responsibility in any conflict by utilizing the Input Box as a model for introspection.

The Input Box contains everything that causes an event to happen. The I-Zone represents everything you bring to the situation: your perception or interpretation of an event, your internal dialogue or self-talk that describes what's happening, and your behavioral response. The They-Zone contains everything in the situation caused by someone or something else: co-workers, fate, circumstance, etc.

The Input Box

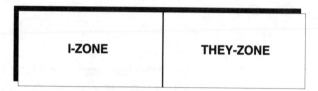

If you are truly self-managed and wish to take responsibility for your own success and happiness, you will focus on the I-Zone in any conflict. The I-Zone is the most critical because it is the only area over which you have direct control. If your intention is to achieve results or become the master of your own fate, you also acknowledge that the *I-Zone can never be empty.* You choose constructive attitudes and behaviors regardless of how others are behaving. If, on the other hand, your true intention is to assign or avoid blame, it is useful to focus on the They-Zone. By doing so, you absolve yourself of any responsibility. But you also create for yourself dependency on outside forces beyond your control. You lose power.

A formula for attaining self-management is to assume that you are always responsible in every situation, even if you don't immediately see how you are. Responsibility is not "duty" or "obligation," nor should it imply blame on your part. Taking responsibility means you acknowledge your choice to respond with maturity and fairness, regardless of circumstances. As a self-managed, responsible person experiencing conflict, you ask yourself the following fundamental questions:

1. "What should be my input to the situation?"

2. "What reactions am I evoking in the other person?"

3. "Is my true intent to resolve the issue and maintain a positive working relationship for the long term?"

4. "Does my behavior reflect this intent?"

The willingness to acknowledge input to any situation is a choice, and it is a prerequisite for assuming responsibility. Assuming responsibility is voluntary: you only do it if you want positive results, freedom, and power in your life.

The Nurse–Physician story described in the previous chapter illustrates that the way you talk and think about situations in your life affects your sense of responsibility. Your internal dialogue makes you more or less responsible. Words or phrases such as "can't" or "I have to" and "I have no choice but to..." facilitate a self-imposed victim, captive, powerless view, and condition you to see difficult situations as problems instead of opportunities for professional growth. Other erroneous thought patterns include: "He makes me feel so mad." "She disappoints me." "That upsets me." Each of these statements suggest that someone else is controlling your emotions. It's *they*, not you.

In his book, *Feeling Good: The New Mood Therapy*, David Beck, M.D. describes a series of "cognitive distortions" that lead to depression and self-defeating behavior.[8] In each case, it is the individual who facilitates her own disappointments based upon her negative interpretation of the events:

1. *All or Nothing Thinking*

This refers to the tendency to see things in black and white terms. For example, if you are criticized by your manager for a mistake or oversight, you conclude, "Now, I'm a total failure." All or nothing thinking forms the basis for perfectionism and causes people to "play it safe," not taking risks for fear of failure.

2. *Overgeneralization*

This refers to seeing a single negative event as a never-ending pattern of defeat. For example, after the manager's criticism, you say to yourself, "Now I've lost complete credibility in her eyes. She thinks I'm incompetent. I hate to see what my appraisal will look like!"

3. *Disqualifying the Positive*

This occurs when you reject positive experiences by insisting they "don't really count." In so doing, you ignore or take for granted any positive experiences and only dwell on the imperfections in the environment. For example, you receive a compliment from your boss and you conclude, "She's just being nice," or your reply is, "Oh, it was nothing really," thereby disqualifying the positive feedback. This type of response only serves to discourage future compliments and facilitates a negative self-fulfilling prophesy.

4. *Jumping to Conclusions*

This is when you make a negative interpretation of an event although there are no facts to support the conclusion. For example, your manager passes you in the hallway and fails to smile or say hello. You conclude, "She's ignoring me so she must not like me any more," or "She's mad at me. What did I do wrong?" or "How rude and ignorant she is!" It could be, however, that she is simply absorbed in thought and doesn't notice you. There was no slight or malice intended. Again, the key to a healthy work relationship is in your interpretation and the meaning you place in the event.

5. *Magnification (Catastrophizing) or Minimization (Discounting)*

This occurs when you inappropriately exaggerate the negative or shrink the positive aspects of any situation. For example, you forget to do something and you say to yourself, "My God, I made a mistake, how terrible, how awful! The word will spread like wildfire! My reputation is ruined." Or, you really accomplished something of significance and you say to yourself, "This is really not a big deal. Anyone could have done this." By magnifying your faults and minimizing your strengths or accomplishments in this way, you set yourself up for low self-esteem.

6.　*Emotional Reasoning*

This occurs when you assume that your negative emotions necessarily reflect the way things really are. You feel it, therefore it must be true. Examples of this include: "I feel guilty; therefore, I must have done something bad." "I feel overwhelmed or helpless; therefore, my problems must be impossible to solve." "I feel inadequate; therefore, I must be worthless." But thinking it doesn't make it so, unless you act on these feelings, thereby causing them to be validated.

7.　*Should Statements*

This occurs when you try to motivate yourself with "shoulds" and "shouldn'ts," as if you have to be psychologically whipped into doing what is right. Albert Ellis refers to this as "musterbation" or a person "shoulding on himself." Likewise, if you direct your should or must statements toward others, you induce unnecessary defensiveness. In either case, you are imposing some external moral standard on yourself or others. The assumption is that, left to your own decision, you would lack the judgment or motivation to do the correct thing.

8.　*Labeling*

This is an extreme form of overgeneralization. Instead of describing and learning from an error you committed, you attach a disabling label onto yourself: "I am a loser." Or when someone else disappoints and irritates you, you say to yourself, "She's a jerk" or "She's stupid and totally incompetent." The problem with labeling is that you can't be equated with any one thing you do. Your life is too complex and changing to pin yourself down in such a fashion. Likewise, when you label someone, you invariably generate hostility, particularly if you express your feelings to the person. Labeling also leads to stereotyping, and while it is tempting to reduce someone to a single characteristic, it is also grossly unfair.

9. *Personalization*

This refers to when you assume blame or guilt for a negative event when there's no basis for doing so. While you are responsible for your own interpretations and behavioral response to any given situation, you're not responsible for someone *else's* attitude or actions. What another person does is ultimately her responsibility. Your actions certainly influence other people, but you cannot control them. Don't give yourself a guilt trip!

If your self-talk reflects any of the above cognitive distortions, recognize that you have a choice to interpret events in a more self-promoting manner. This requires that you continuously challenge the validity of your initial perceptions. These perceptions help create either positive or negative feelings, which in turn, influence your behavioral responses.

▲

Dysfunctional Attitudes
Contributing to Job Frustration

Four examples of dysfunctional attitudes that contribute to job frustration:

1. *Making yourself feel indispensable*
   "If I'm not there, the unit will fall apart.
   People depend on me!"

Comment:

Of course, you are valuable but no one, including yourself, is indispensable. If for some uncontrollable circumstance, you were forced to miss work for a sustained period of time, the unit would survive. When you come to believe that other people could not succeed unless you are ever-present, you assume unnecessary burdens. You need to think about your own needs and if you don't, you will burn yourself out and be unable to provide a valuable service in the long run.

2. *Owning Other People's Problems*
   "When I become aware of someone's troubles,
   I feel a duty to help them out even if it results
   in my own inconvenience."

Comment:

This attitude facilitates a hyper-sense of personal responsibility or co-dependency, especially if you focus on meeting the needs of others to the point of self-neglect. Sometimes you can get too personally involved in others' problems. By taking on their burdens or by providing unsolicited advice, you then take responsibility for the outcome of the person's decisions and inadvertently place the proverbial monkey on your shoulders.

3. *Doing It All Yourself*
"If you want something to be done right, do it yourself!"

Comment:
This attitude facilitates a false sense of independence making it difficult for you to ask for help, delegate, or share responsibility. Your on-the-job survival is contingent upon learning the skills of informal negotiation and delegation. You simply cannot do it all or be all things to all people. You also save much time and lessen aggravation in the long run when you empower others to take responsibility. Delegating is not dumping. But if done properly, you develop others' skills, a sense of responsibility, and teamwork within the unit.

continued...

Dysfunctional Attitudes
Contributing to Job Frustration

...continued

4. *Avoiding Conflict at All Costs*
"If I play it smart, I can side-step controversy and conflicts, thereby making my life more peaceful."

Comment:
Conflict is not bad. Conflict is not good. Conflict just *is*. How you deal with conflict can be very positive or counterproductive. The myth that conflict is inherently negative may cause you to escape from a confrontation that is both necessary and inevitable. Furthermore, not all conflict can be prevented. You must learn, therefore, how to assertively express your needs and how to set limits when someone is not fighting fairly with you.

Every conflict is an opportunity to test your beliefs, learn from different perspectives, and to practice assertive self-management. Don't look for unnecessary conflict in your life, but deal with it when it exists. Approach people directly, honestly and respectfully. By doing so, you improve the odds of leading a productive and satisfying work life.

Notes:

Other Irrational Thoughts

Excerpts from *A New Guide to Rational Living*[9]

1. It is a *dire* necessity to be loved and approved of.

2. I *should* be *thoroughly* competent, adequate and achieving in *all* possible respects.

3. If things do not go (or stay) the way I very much want them to, it would be *awful, catastrophic or terrible!*

4. Unhappiness is *externally* caused and I *cannot* control it (unless I control the other person).

5. It is *easier* to avoid responsibility and difficulties than to face them.

6. I have a *right* to be dependent, and people (or someone) should be strong enough to rely on (or take care of me).

7. My early childhood experiences *must* continue to control me and determine my emotions and behavior!

8. I *should* become upset over other people's problems and behavior.

9. There is invariably one right, precise, and *perfect* solution and it would be *terrible* or *catastrophic* if this perfect solution is not found.

10. The world (and especially other people) should be fair, and justice (or mercy) *must* triumph.

We have to face the fact that either all of us are going to die together or we are going to learn to live together.
And if we are to live together we have to talk.

Eleanor Roosevelt

▲

Chapter 13

EPILOGUE

You Are Not Alone

There are valuable resources within your organization to help you improve your job performance or satisfaction. Below is a checklist of resources offered by many employers. Check the ones that are available to you.

❑   Manager's availability and willingness to discuss the problem with you if it's addressed in constructive manner

❑   Neutral, objective third party (other than manager) to help you sort out the problem on a confidential basis

❑   Formal grievance procedure

❑   Career counseling and/or job transfer opportunities

❑   Continuing education and/or job training opportunities

❑   Task force or committee membership opportunities

❑   Social and recreational activities

❑   Others:

It is your responsibility to identify and use all available resources that will improve your job performance and satisfaction. Before you ask for help, however, ask yourself: What really is the issue and what are my specific expectations? What constructive role can I play in solving the particular problem? Are my expectations realistic? Am I open to any suggestions for change?

In most cases, you should initially try to solve the problem *within* your own work area by discussing the issue directly with the person with whom you're having the difficulty. If necessary, seek assistance from your manager. If the problem cannot be solved on this level, use organizational resources available to you outside your department.

In addition to the use of formal organizational resources, it is important to develop an informal support system of friends and professional colleagues. These individuals can serve as a confidential sounding board to help you clarify your work problem and provide you with guidance on how to constructively manage yourself. But ultimately, these people cannot solve the problem for you. Nor should these discussions serve as a substitute for direct, honest and respectful communication with the person you are experiencing difficulty. By using the strategies described in this book, the chances are good that you can either effectively resolve the problem or make the necessary attitudinal adjustments that will facilitate your job success and satisfaction.

The power of self-management is great. Yes, you are only one person, but one person can make a difference. You can't do everything, but you can always do something. And what you can do, you should do. Common sense is simply the knack of seeing things as they are and doing things as they ought to be done in a responsible and ethical manner. Theodore Roosevelt said, "Do what you can, with what you have, where you are." James Baldwin said, "Not everything that is faced can be changed, but nothing can be changed unless it is faced."

Self-management on the job is a commitment to stretch emotionally, intellectually and behaviorally in pursuit of goals that are worthy of accomplishment. To tend unfailingly or unflinchingly to an idea or task, having confidence in yourself, and applying yourself with all your might to your work, *is* the secret to job success and fulfillment. Achievement is not an ethical duty imposed upon someone from above. It is, in the last analysis, a manifestation of your deepest desire that your life will have significance. Every form of success and happiness is self-motivated. And, every great achievement has its source in self-management.

▲

Enriching Yourself on the Job

If you're interested in gaining a greater measure of job success and satisfaction, identify ways you can get involved in issues that will utilize your talents. Complete the following exercise and follow through with an action plan.

Activities I would like to get involved in where I can make a valuable contribution:

Person I have to convince:

▲

- _____

- _____

- _____

- _____

- _____

- _____

- _____

- _____

- _____

- _____

Develop a plan of action to "market" your role in these activities or, if appropriate, determine what additional training or education will be required to justify your involvement in these activities

▲

Characteristics of a Self-Managed Employee

- Appreciates the work environment yet tries to continuously improve it. Strives toward greater efficiency, to make an operation neater, simpler, faster, safer, more fool-proof, with less expense, time and effort.

- Views work as important, even critical, and truly values the opportunity to serve others.

- Enjoys happy endings, good completions.

- Prefers peace and pleasantries over interpersonal and group conflict.

- Demonstrates the capacity to work independently and follow through on tasks.

- Retains a steadiness of purpose in spite of time pressures and limited resources.

- Searches for practical solutions to problems.

- Looks for the latest in new ideas and developments that apply to the workplace.

- Avoids the obvious and advances creative approaches to challenging situations.

- Enjoys situations that stretch skills and imagination.

- Supports a good suggestion in the common interest of the team, regardless who sponsored the idea.

- Works well with a wide range of people, including those with different personalities and work styles.

- Provides constructive criticism without attacking others by "packaging" comments in a sensitive manner.

- Maintains control during frustrating situations.

- Responds to change in an open and flexible manner and works for its success in spite of personal misgivings.

- Brings a touch of professionalism to any job.

Notes:

To know and not to do is not to know.

Buddha

▲

Setting Yourself Up For Success

Now that you have had an opportunity to review effective self-management strategies for achieving success in your healthcare career, please complete this Individual Commitment Form.

One technique that I am going to choose to be more self-managed is:

because

I will use this behavior whenever

What do I need help on? Whom can I ask for help? What additional information would be helpful?

What are the biggest barriers I have to guard against, and how can I overcome them?

FOOTNOTES

1. Katz, Stan J. & Liv, Aimee E., *Success Trap*, New York, N.Y., A Dell Publishing, 1991.

2. Frankl, Viktor E., *Man's Search for Meaning: An Introduction to Logotherapy*, New York, N.Y., Washington Square Press, Inc., 1969.

3. ibid.

4. ibid.

5. *American Journal of Psychology*, Vol. 42, (pp.444–5), "A New Ambiguous Figure," E.G. Boring, 1930.

6. Heider, John, *The Tao of Leadership: Leadership Strategies for a New Age*, New York, N.Y., Bantam Books, 1986.

7. Covey, Steven R., *The Seven Habits of Highly Effective People*, New York, N.Y., Simon & Schuster, 1989.

8. Beck, David, M.D., *Feeling Good: The New Mood Therapy*, New York, N.Y., A Signet Book, 1980.

9. Ellis, Albert & Harper, R.A., *A New Guide to Rational Living*, Englewood Cliffs, N.J., Prentice Hall, 1975.

Quotations throughout the book from:

Phillips, Bob, *Powerful Thinking for Powerful Living*, Eugene, Oregon, Harvest House Publishers, 1991.

Partnow, Elaine, Ed., *The Quotable Woman*, Garden City, N.Y., Anchor Press, 1978.

Additional copies of *The Power of Self-Management* can be ordered by mail from the publisher. Enclose check or money order of $10.25 per book (price includes shipping and handling) to:

Canoe Press
P.O. Box 174
Oak Park, IL 60303

Copies of Michael H. Cohen's other book, *On-The-Job-Survival,* can also be ordered by mail from Canoe Press by enclosing a check or money order of $9.25.

Inquire about special rates for quantity orders of either book by calling (708) 386-1968 or by writing to the address above.

Please send me _____ copies of
The Power of Self-Management @ $10.25 each
(includes postage and handling)

Enclosed is my check or money order for $_____
(no cash or C.O.D.'s please)

Name _____

Organization_____

Address _____

City _____ State _____ Zip _____

Canoe Press. Oak Park. Illinois